SIMPLY CROCKPOT 2022

EASY AND HEALTHY RECIPES FOR BEGINNERS

SANDRA SUTTON

Table of Contents

Chicken With Noodles, Slow Cooker

INGREDIENTS

-
2 teaspoons chicken bouillon granules or base

-
1 tablespoon chopped fresh parsley

-
3/4 teaspoon poultry seasoning

-
1/3 cup. diced Canadian bacon or smoked ham

-
2 to 3 carrots, thinly sliced

-
2 ribs celery, thinly sliced

-
1 small onion, thinly sliced

-
1/4 cup. water

-
1 broiler-fryer chicken (about 3 pounds), cut up

-
1 (10 3/4 oz.) can condensed cheddar cheese soup

-
1 tablespoon all purpose flour

- 1 (16 oz.) pkg. wide egg noodles, cooked and drained

- 2 tablespoons sliced pimento

- 2 tablespoons grated Parmesan cheese

PREPARATION

1.
In a small bowl, combine chicken bouillon or base, chopped parsley, and poultry seasoning; set aside.

2.
In slow cooker, layer Canadian bacon or ham, carrots, celery and onion. Add water.

3.
Remove skin and excess fat from chicken; rinse and pat dry. Place half the chicken in slow cooker. Sprinkle with half of the reserved seasoning mixture. Top with remaining chicken and sprinkle with remaining seasoning mixture.

4.
Stir soup and flour together and spoon over the chicken; do not stir.

5.
Cover and cook on HIGH for 3 to 3 1/2 hours or on low for 6 to 8 hours, or until chicken is tender and juices from chicken run clear when cut along the bone and vegetables are tender.

6.
Put hot cooked noodles in a shallow 2 to 2 1/2 quart broiler proof serving dish. Arrange chicken over the noodles. Stir soup mixture and vegetables in crockpot until blended. Spoon vegetables and some of the liquid over chicken. Sprinkle with sliced pimiento and Parmesan cheese.

7.

Broil 4 to 6 inches from heat source for 5 to 8 minutes, or until lightly browned.

8.

Garnish with parsley sprig if desired.

9.

Alpine chicken recipe serves 4 to 6.

Chicken with Onions

INGREDIENTS

- 4 large onions, sliced thinly

- 5 cloves garlic, minced

- 1/4 cup lemon juice

- 1 teaspoon salt

- 1/4 teaspoon cayenne pepper (or more if you like)

- 4 to 6 frozen boneless chicken breasts, no need to thaw

- hot cooked rice

PREPARATION

1.
Put all ingredients except rice in Crock Pot. Mix well. Cook for 4 to 6 hours on LOW, or until chicken is cooked through and still tender.

2.
Serve over rice.

Chicken With Parsley Dumplings

INGREDIENTS

- 4 to 6 chicken breast halves, skin removed

- 1 dash each salt, pepper, dried leaf thyme, ground marjoram and paprika

- 1 large onion, sliced, divided

- 2 leeks, sliced

- 4 carrots, cut large chunks

- 1 garlic clove, minced

- 1 cup chicken broth

- 1 tablespoon cornstarch

- 1 can (10 3/4 ounces) condensed cream of chicken soup

- 1/2 cup dry white wine

- Dumplings

- 1 cup Bisquick

- 8 tablespoons milk

- 1 teaspoon dried parsley flakes

- dash salt

- dash pepper

- dash paprika

PREPARATION

1.
Sprinkle salt, pepper, thyme, marjoram, and paprika on chicken. In bottom of crockpot, place half of the onion slices, leeks, and carrots. Arrange chicken on vegetables. Sprinkle minced garlic over the chicken then top with remaining onion slices. Dissolve 1 tablespoon cornstarch in 1 cup of chicken broth then combine with the cream of chicken soup and wine. Cook on HIGH for about 3 hours or on LOW for about 6 hours (If cooking on LOW, turn to HIGH when dumplings are added).

2.
Chicken should be tender, but not dry.

3.
Dumplings: Mix together 1 cup bisquick, about 8 tablespoon milk, parsley, salt, pepper, and paprika; form into balls and place on top of the chicken mixture the last 35 to 45 minutes of cooking.

4.
Serves 4 to 6.

Chicken With Pearl Onions and Mushrooms

INGREDIENTS

- 4 to 6 boneless chicken breast halves, cut in 1-inch chunks

- 1 can (10 3/4 ounces) cream of chicken or cream of chicken and mushroom soup

- 8 ounces sliced mushrooms

- 1 bag (16 ounces) frozen pearl onions

- salt and pepper, to taste

- parsley, chopped, for garnish

PREPARATION

1.
Wash chicken and pat dry. Cut into chunks about 1/2 to 1-inch and put in a large bowl. Add the soup, mushrooms, and onions; stir to combine. Spray the slow cooker insert with cooking spray.

2.
Spoon the chicken mixture into the crockpot and sprinkle with salt and pepper.

3.
Cover and cook on LOW for 6 to 8 hours, stirring about halfway through the cooking time, if possible.

4.

Garnish with fresh chopped parsley, if desired, and serve over hot cooked rice or with potatoes.

5.

Serves 4 to 6.

Chicken With Pineapple

INGREDIENTS

- 1 to 1 1/2 pounds chicken tenders, cut in 1-inch pieces

- 2/3 cup pineapple preserves

- 1 tablespoon plus 1 teaspoon teriyaki sauce

- 2 cloves garlic sliced thinly

- 1 tablespoon dried minced onion (or 1 bunch fresh green onions, chopped)

- 1 tablespoon lemon juice

- 1/2 teaspoon ground ginger

- dash cayenne, to taste

- 1 package (10 oz) sugar snap peas, thawed

PREPARATION

1.

Place chicken pieces in slow cooker/Crock Pot.

2.

Combine preserves, teriyaki sauce, garlic, onion, lemon juice, ginger, and cayenne; stir well. Spoon over chicken, toss to coat.

3.

Cover and cook on low 6 to 7 hours. Add peas last 30 minutes.

4.

Serves 4.

Chicken-Rice Casserole

INGREDIENTS

-
4 to 6 large chicken breasts, boneless, skinned

-
1 can cream of chicken soup

-
1 can cream of celery soup

-
1 can cream of mushroom soup

-
1/2 cup diced celery

-
1 to 1 1/2 cups converted rice

PREPARATION

1.

In slow cooker, combine 3 cans of soup and rice. Place the chicken on top of the mixture, then add the diced celery. Cook for 3 hours on high or about 6 to 7 hours on low.

2.

Makes 4 to 6 servings.

Chili Chicken

INGREDIENTS

- 6 boneless chicken breast halves, cut in 1-inch pieces

- 1 cup chopped onion

- 1 cup chopped bell pepper

- 2 garlic cloves

- 2 tbsp. vegetable oil

- 2 cans Mexican stewed tomatoes (approx. 15 ounces each)

- 1 can chili beans

- 2/3 cup picante sauce

- 1 teaspoon. chili powder

- 1 teaspoon. cumin

- 1/2 teaspoon. Salt

PREPARATION

1.

Saute chicken, onion, pepper, garlic in vegetable oil until vegetables are wilted. Transfer to slow cooker; add remaining ingredients. Cover and cook on LOW for 4 to 6 hours. Serve with rice.

2.

Serves 4 to 6.

Chinese-Style Chicken and Vegetables

INGREDIENTS

- 1 to 1 1/2 pounds chicken breast tenders, boneless

- 2 cups coarsely chopped cabbage

- 1 medium onion, cut in large chunks

- 1 medium red bell pepper, cut in large chunks

- 1 packet Kikkoman Chicken Salad Seasoning

- 1 tablespoon red wine vinegar

- 2 teaspoons honey

- 1 tablespoon soy sauce

- 1 cup frozen mixed oriental vegetables

- 2 tablespoons cornstarch

- 1 tablespoon cold water

PREPARATION

1.

Cut chicken into 1 1/2-inch pieces. Place first 8 ingredients in slow cooker; mix well. Cover and cook on low for 5 to 7 hours. Stir cornstarch and cold water together; add with vegetables and cook for 30 to 45 minutes longer, until vegetables are tender.

2.

Serves 4 to 6.

Cornish Game Hens with Rice

INGREDIENTS

- 2 Cornish game hens

- 1/2 cup chicken broth

- Salt and lemon pepper to taste

- hot boiled rice

PREPARATION

1.

Place Cornish hens in the slow cooker (brown hens in a lightly greased skillet first, if desired). Add chicken broth. Sprinkle the hens with salt and lemon pepper. Cook on LOW setting for 7 to 9 hours. Remove hens and skim fat; thicken juices with a mixture of 1 1/2 tablespoons of cornstarch and 1 tablespoon cold water. Serve with hot cooked rice. Serves 2.

Cornish Hens with Raisin Sauce

INGREDIENTS

-
1 package (6 ounces) stuffing mix, prepared as directed

-
4 Cornish game hens

-
salt and pepper

-
.

-
Raisin Sauce

-
1 jar (10 ounces) currant jelly

-
1/2 cup raisins

-
1/4 cup butter

-
1 tablespoon lemon juice

-
1/4 teaspoon allspice

PREPARATION

1.

Stuff hens with prepared stuffing; sprinkle with salt and pepper. Place trivet or crumpled piece of heavy-duty foil in slow cooker, to keep hens from sitting in juices. If you're using a deep and narrow crockpot, put Cornish hens in neck-side down. In a 1-quart saucepan combine jelly, raisins, butter, lemon juice and allspice. Cook over low heat, stirring, until hot and simmering. Brush some of the sauce on hens in the crockpot.

2.

Keep remaining sauce in refrigerator until serving time. Cover and cook on LOW for 5 to 7 hours, basting once about an hour before done. Bring remaining sauce to a boil and spoon over hens at serving time.

3.

Makes 4 servings.

Country Captain Chicken Breasts

INGREDIENTS

- 2 medium-size Granny Smith apples, cored and diced (unpeeled)

- 1/4 cup finely chopped onion

- 1 small green bell pepper, seeded and finely chopped

- 3 cloves garlic, minced

- 2 tablespoons raisins or currants

- 2 to 3 teaspoons curry powder

- 1 teaspoon ground ginger

- 1/4 teaspoon ground red pepper, or to taste

- 1 can (about 14 1/2 oz.) diced tomatoes

- 6 boneless chicken breast halves, skin removed

- 1/2 cup chicken broth

- 1 cup long-grain converted white rice

-

1 pound medium to large shrimp, shelled and deveined, uncooked, optional

-

1/3 cup slivered almonds

-

kosher salt

-

Chopped parsley

PREPARATION

1.

In a 4- to 6-quart slow cooker, combine diced apples, onion, bell pepper, garlic, golden raisins or currants, curry powder, ginger, and ground red pepper; stir in tomatoes.

2.

Arrange the chicken over the tomato mixture, overlapping pieces slightly. Pour chicken broth over the chicken breast halves. Cover and cook on LOW until chicken is very tender when pierced with a fork, about 4 to 6 hours.

3.

Remove chicken to a warm plate, cover lightly, and keep warm in a 200° F oven or warming drawer.

4.

Stir the rice into cooking liquid. Increase temperature to high; cover and cook, stirring once or twice, until rice is almost tender, about 35 minutes. Stir in shrimp, if using; cover and cook for about 15 minutes longer, until shrimp are opaque in center; cut to test.

5.

Meanwhile, toast almonds in a small nonstick frying pan over medium heat until golden brown, stirring occasionally. Set aside.

6.

To serve the dish, season rice mixture to taste with salt. Mound in a warm serving dish; arrange chicken on top. Sprinkle with parsley and almonds.

Country Chicken and Mushrooms

INGREDIENTS

-
1 jar country gravy

-
4 to 6 chicken breasts

-
8 ounces sliced mushrooms

-
salt and pepper to taste

PREPARATION

1.
Combine all ingredients; cover and cook on low for 6 to 7 hours. Serve with rice or noodles.

2.
Serves 4 to 6.

Country Club Chicken

INGREDIENTS

- 5 apples, peeled, cored & chopped

- 6 to 8 green onions, with green, sliced

- 1 lb chicken thighs, deboned, skinned, all fat removed, cut into 2-inch cubes

- 6 to 8 ounces sliced Swiss cheese

- 1 can (10 1/2 ounces) cream of chicken soup, well blended with 1/4 cup milk

- 1 box (6 ounces) Pepperidge Farm Stuffing with Apples and Raisins, or use your favorite stuffing mix

- 1/4 cup melted butter

- 3/4 cup apple juice

PREPARATION

1.
Layer ingredients in 3-1/2 to 5-quart slow cooker in same order as above. Pour soup mixture over cheese layer, butter over stuffing and finally drizzle with the apple juice, making sure that liquid moistens all of the bread.

2.
Cover and cook on HIGH for 1 hour and on LOW for another 4 to 5 hours.

3.
Rose-Marie's Note:

4.
We ate it without anything but since it makes a wonderful sauce and the stuffing sort of disappears into the dish, I recommend serving it with plain rice.

Cranberry Chicken

INGREDIENTS

- 4 to 6 boneless chicken breast halves, skin removed

- 1 can whole cranberry sauce

- 2/3 cup chili sauce

- 2 tablespoons cider vinegar

- 2 tablespoons brown sugar

- 1 package dry (Lipton) golden onion soup mix

PREPARATION

1.
Place chicken breasts in the slow cooker/Crock Pot. Combine remaining ingredients; add to the slow cooker/Crock Pot, coating chicken well. Cover and cook on low 6 to 8 hours.

2.
Serves 4 to 6.

Cranberry Chicken II

INGREDIENTS

- 2 pounds boneless chicken breasts, skin removed

- 1/2 cup chopped onion

- 2 teaspoons vegetable oil

- 2 teaspoons salt

- 1/2 teaspoon ground cinnamon

- 1/4 teaspoon ground ginger

- 1/8 teaspoon ground nutmeg

- dash ground allspice

- 1 cup orange juice

- 2 teaspoons finely grated orange peel

- 2 cups fresh or frozen cranberries

- 1/4 cup brown sugar

PREPARATION

1.

Brown chicken pieces and onion in oil; sprinkle with salt.

2.

Add browned chicken, onions and other ingredients to crock pot.

3.

Cover and cook on LOW 5 1/2 to 7 hours.

4.

If desired, thicken juices near the end of cooking time with a mixture of about 2 tablespoons cornstarch combined with 2 tablespoons cold water.

Cream Cheese Chicken

INGREDIENTS

- 3 to 3 1/2 pounds chicken parts

- 2 tablespoons melted butter

- salt and pepper, to taste

- 2 tablespoons dry Italian salad dressing

- 1 can (10 3/4 ounces) cream of mushroom soup

- 8 ounces cream cheese, cut into cubes

- 1/2 cup dry white wine

- 1 tablespoon chopped onion

PREPARATION

1.
Brush chicken with butter and sprinkle with salt and pepper. Place in a slow cooked and sprinkle dry dressing mix over all.

2.
Cover and cook on low for 6 to 7 hours, or until the chicken is tender and cooked through.

3.

About 45 minutes before done, mix soup, cream cheese, wine, and onion in a small saucepan. Cook until bubbly and smooth.

4.

Pour over the chicken and cover and cook 30 to 45 minutes longer.

5.

Serve chicken with sauce.

6.

Serves 4 to 6.

Creamy Chicken and Artichokes

INGREDIENTS

-
2 to 3 cups cooked, cubed chicken

-
2 cups frozen artichoke quarters or 1 can (about 15 ounces), drained

-
2 ounces chopped pimiento, drained

-
1 jar (16 ounces) Alfredo sauce

-
1 teaspoon chicken base or bouillon

-
1/2 teaspoon dried basil

-
1/2 teaspoon garlic granules or powder

-
1 teaspoon dried parsley, optional

-
salt and pepper to taste

-
8 ounces spaghetti, cooked and drained, optional

PREPARATION

1.

I poach about a pound of chicken tenders in a little lemon and garlic seasoned water, but you can use cooked chicken breasts or leftover chicken. Combine all ingredients in the crockpot; cover and cook on low for 4 to 6 hours. Stir in hot cooked pasta or use as a sauce for rice or pasta. This slow cooker chicken and artichokes recipe serves 4 to 6.

Creamy Italian Chicken

INGREDIENTS

-

4 boneless skinless chicken breast halves

-

1 envelope Italian salad dressing mix

-

1/3 cup water

-

1 package (8 ozs.) cream cheese, softened

-

1 can (10 3/4 ozs.) condensed cream of chicken soup, undiluted

-

1 can (4 ozs.) mushroom stems and pieces, drained

-

Hot cooked rice or noodles

PREPARATION

1.

Place the chicken breast halves in a slow cooker. Combine salad dressing
mix and water; pour over chicken. Cover and cook on LOW for 3 hours. In a
small mixing bowl, whisk together cream cheese and soup until blended. Stir
in mushrooms. Pour cream cheese mixture over chicken. Cook 1 to 3 hours
longer or until chicken juices run clear. Serve Italian chicken with rice or hot
cooked noodles.

2.

Serves 4.

Creole Chicken

INGREDIENTS

- 1 frying chicken, cut up, about 3 pounds chicken pieces

- 1 green bell pepper, chopped

- 6 green onions, about 1 bunch, chopped

- 1 can (14.5 ounces) tomatoes, undrained, cut up

- 1 can (6 ounces) tomato paste

- 4 ounces cooked diced ham

- 1 teaspoon salt

- several drops of bottled hot pepper sauce, such as Tabasco

- 1/2 pound sliced smoked sausage, andouille, kielbasa, etc.

- 3 cups cooked rice

PREPARATION

1.

In slow cooker, combine the chicken, pepper, onions, tomatoes, tomato paste, ham, salt, and pepper sauce.

2.

Cover and cook on low for 6 hours. Turn control to high and add sausage and cooked rice. Cover and cook on high for 20 minutes longer.

Creole Chicken With Sausage

INGREDIENTS

- 1 1/2 pounds boneless chicken thighs, cut into chunks

- 12 ounces smoked andouille sausage, cut in 1- to 2-inch lengths

- 1 cup chopped onions

- 3/4 cup chicken broth or water

- 1 can (14.5 ounces) diced tomatoes

- 1 can (6 ounces) tomato paste

- 2 teaspoons Cajun or Creole seasoning

- dash cayenne pepper, to taste

- 1 green bell pepper, chopped

- salt and pepper, to taste

- hot cooked white or brown rice or cooked drained spaghetti

PREPARATION

1.

In a slow cooker, combine the chicken thigh pieces, andouille sausage pieces, chopped onions, broth or water, tomatoes (with their juices), tomato paste, Creole seasoning, and cayenne pepper.

2.

Cover and cook the chicken and sausage mixture on LOW for 6 to 7 hours. Add the chopped green bell pepper about an hour before the dish is done. Taste and add salt and pepper, as needed.

3.

Serve this flavorful chicken and sausage dish over hot boiled rice, or serve it with spaghetti or angel hair pasta.

4.

Serves 6.

Crock Pot Chicken and Artichokes

INGREDIENTS

- 3 pounds chicken pieces, broiler-fryer, cut up

- salt, to taste

- 1/2 teaspoon pepper

- 1/2 teaspoon paprika

- 1 tablespoon butter

- 2 jars marinated artichoke, hearts; reserve marinade

- 1 can (4 ounces) mushrooms, drained

- 2 tablespoons quick-cooking tapioca

- 1/2 cup chicken broth

- 3 tablespoons dry sherry or more chicken broth

- 1/2 teaspoon dried tarragon

PREPARATION

1.

Wash chicken and pat dry. Season chicken with salt, pepper, and paprika. In a large skillet over medium heat, brown chicken in butter and the reserved marinade from artichokes.

2.

Place mushrooms and artichoke hearts in bottom of slow cooker. Sprinkle with tapioca. Add the browned chicken pieces. Pour in chicken broth and sherry. Add tarragon. Cover and cook on LOW for 7 to 8 hours, or cook on HIGH for 3 1/2 to 4 1/2 hours.

3.

Serves 4.

Crock Pot Chicken And Dressing

INGREDIENTS

- 4 boneless chicken breast halves, without skin+

- salt and freshly ground black pepper, to taste

- 4 slices swiss cheese

- 1 can (10 3/4 ounces) condensed cream of chicken soup

- 1 can (10 3/4 ounces) condensed cream of mushroom soup or cream of celery

- 1 cup chicken broth

- 1/4 cup milk

- 3 cups herb seasoned stuffing crumbs

- 1/2 cup melted butter

PREPARATION

1.

Season chicken breasts with salt and pepper and place them in the slow cooker. Pour chicken broth over chicken breasts. Put one slice of Swiss cheese on each breast.

2.

Combine both cans of soup and the milk in a bowl; blend well. Pour the soup mixture over the chicken. Sprinkle stuffing mix over all. Drizzle melted butter over the stuffing layer.

3.

Cover and cook on low for 5 to 7 hours.

4.

Note: Chicken breasts are very lean and become dry when overcooked.

5.

Depending on your slow cooker, the chicken might be done perfectly in 4 hours or less. For the longer cooking time, try the recipe with boneless chicken thighs.

Crock Pot Chicken Enchilada Hot Dish

INGREDIENTS

- 9 corn tortillas, 6-inch

- 1 can (12 to 16 ounces) whole kernel corn with peppers, drained

- 2 to 3 cups cooked diced chicken

- 1 teaspoon chili powder

- 1/4 teaspoon ground black pepper

- 1/2 teaspoon salt, or to taste

- 1 can (4 ounces) chopped green chile peppers, mild

- 2 cups shredded Mexican blend cheese or mild Cheddar cheese

- 2 cans (10 ounces each) enchilada sauce

- 1 can (15 ounces) black beans, rinsed and drained

- guacamole and sour cream

PREPARATION

1.

Spray slow cooker with nonstick cooking spray.

2.

Place 3 tortillas in bottom of slow cooker.

3.

Top tortillas with the corn, half of the chicken, about half of the seasonings, and half of the chile peppers.

4.

Sprinkle with half of the shredded cheese and pour about 3/4 cup of enchilada sauce over the cheese.

5.

Repeat with 3 more tortillas, the black beans, remaining chicken, seasonings, chile peppers, and cheese.

1.

Top with remaining tortillas and enchilada sauce.

2.

Cover and cook on LOW setting for 5 to 6 hours.

3.

Serve with guacamole and sour cream.

4.

Serves 6 to 8.

Crock Pot Chicken Enchiladas

INGREDIENTS

- 1 large can (19 ounces) enchilada sauce

- 6 boneless chicken breast halves

- 2 cans cream of chicken soup

- 1 small can sliced black olives

- 1/2 cup chopped onion

- 1 can (4 ounces) chopped mild chile peppers

- 16 to 20 corn tortillas

- 16 ounces shredded sharp Cheddar cheese

PREPARATION

1.
Cook chicken and shred. Mix soup, olives, chile peppers, and onions. Cut tortillas in wedges. Layer Crock Pot with sauce, tortillas, soup mix, chicken and cheese all the way to top, ending with cheese on top. Cover and cook on LOW for 5 to 7 hours.

2.
Serves 8 to 10

Crock Pot Chicken Tortillas

INGREDIENTS

- 4 cups cooked chicken shredded or cut into bite-size pieces

- 1 can cream of chicken soup

- 1/2 c. green chile salsa

- 2 tbsp. quick cooking tapioca

- 1 med. onion, chopped

- 1 1/2 c. shredded cheese

- 12 to 15 corn tortillas

- Black olives

- 1 tomato, chopped

- 2 tablespoons chopped green onion

- sour cream for garnish

PREPARATION

1.

Combine chicken with soup, chile salsa, and tapioca. Line bottom of Crock Pot with 3 corn tortillas, torn into bite size pieces. Add 1/3 of the chicken mixture. Sprinkle with 1/3 of the onion and 1/3 of the grated cheese. Repeat layers of tortillas topped with chicken mixture, onions and cheese. Cover and cook on low 6 to 8 hours or high for 3 hours. Garnish with sliced black olives, chopped tomatoes, green onion, and sour cream, if desired.

Crockpot Cassoulet

INGREDIENTS

- 1 pound dry navy beans, rinsed

- 4 cups water

- 4 boneless chicken breast halves without skin, cut in 1-inch pieces

- 8 ounces cooked ham, cut in 1-inch pieces

- 3 large carrots, thinly sliced

- 1 cup chopped onion

- 1/2 cup sliced celery

- 1/4 cup firmly packed brown sugar

- 1/2 teaspoon salt

- 1/4 teaspoon dry mustard

- 1/4 teaspoon pepper

- 1 can (8 ounces) tomato sauce

-
2 tablespoons molasses

PREPARATION

2.

In

Dutch oven or large kettle, soak beans overnight in 4 cups water.

3.

Cover and simmer beans over low heat for about 1 1/2 hours, until tender, adding a little more water as necessary.

4.

Put the beans and liquid in the crockpot. Add remaining ingredients; mix well.

5.

Cover and cook on LOW for 7 to 9 hours, until vegetables are tender.

6.

Serves 6 to 8.

Crockpot Chicken and Herb Dumplings

INGREDIENTS

- 3 pounds chicken pieces, skin removed

- salt and pepper

- 1/4 cup chopped onions

- 10 small white onions

- 2 cloves garlic, minced

- 1/4 teaspoon ground marjoram

- 1/2 teaspoon dried leaf thyme, crumbled

- 1 bay leaf

- 1/2 cup dry white wine

- 1 cup dairy sour cream

- 1 cup biscuit mix

- 1 tablespoon chopped parsley

-
6 tablespoons milk

PREPARATION

1.

Sprinkle chicken with salt and pepper, place in slow cooker or crockpot. Put all onions into pot. Add garlic, marjoram, thyme, bay leaf and wine. Cover and cook on low 5 to 6 hours. Remove bay leaf. Stir in sour cream. Increase heat to high and combine biscuit mix with parsley. Stir milk into biscuit mix until well moistened. Drop dumplings from teaspoon around edge of pot. Cover and continue to cook on high for 30 minutes longer, until dumplings are cooked.

Crockpot Chicken Barbecue

INGREDIENTS

-
2 boneless, skinless chicken breasts

-
1 1/2 cups tomato ketchup

-
3 tablespoons brown sugar

-
1 tablespoon Worcestershire sauce

-
1 tablespoon soy sauce

-
1 tablespoon cider vinegar

-
1 teaspoon ground red hot pepper flakes, or to taste

-
1/2 teaspoon garlic powder

PREPARATION

1.

Combine all ingredients for the sauce in the slow cooker. Add the chicken; turn to coat thoroughly with the sauce.

2.

Cook on high 3 to 4 hours, or until chicken is fully cooked. Shred or chop chicken, and return it to the sauce in the pot. Mix well so all the pieces are coated.

3.

You can keep the slow cooker on low to keep the chicken warm for serving on hard rolls.

4.

Delicious!

Crockpot Chicken Barbecue

INGREDIENTS

- 1 frying chicken, cut up or quartered

- 1 can condensed tomato soup

- 3/4 c. chopped onion

- 1/4 c. vinegar

- 3 tbsp. brown sugar

- 1 tbsp. Worcestershire sauce

- 1/2 tsp. salt

- 1/4 tsp. sweet basil

- pinch thyme

PREPARATION

1.

Place chicken in slow cooker. Combine all other ingredients and pour over chicken. Cover tightly and cook on LOW for 6 to 8 hours. Serves 4.

Crockpot Chicken Chili

INGREDIENTS

- 2 cups great northern dried beans, soaked overnight

- 3 cups boiling water

- 1 cup chopped onion

- 2 garlic cloves, minced

- 2 to 3 canned jalapeno peppers, chopped (pickled is fine)

- 1 tablespoon ground cumin

- 1 teaspoon chili powder

- 1 to 1 1/2 pounds boneless chicken breasts, cut into 1-inch pieces

- 2 small zucchini or summer squash, cubed

- 1 can (12 to 15 ounces) whole kernel corn, drained

- 1/2 cup sour cream

- 2 1/4 teaspoons salt

- 1 tablespoon lime juice

- 1/4 cup chopped fresh cilantro, and some for garnish, if desired

- 1 tomato, chopped, for garnish, or halved cherry tomatoes

- sour cream for garnish

PREPARATION

1.

Combine beans and boiling water in slow-cooker. Let stand while preparing other ingredients. Add chopped onion, minced garlic, jalapeno pepper, cumin and chili powder to the crockpot. Place chicken on top. Add cubed squash to the pot. Cover and cook on low heat for 7 to 8 hours or until beans are tender. Stir in corn, sour cream, salt, lime juice and chopped cilantro. Spoon into bowls. Garnish with a spoonful of sour cream, chopped tomato and chopped fresh cilantro, if desired.

Crockpot Chicken Chow Mein

INGREDIENTS

-

1 1/2 pounds boneless chicken breasts, cut into 1-inch chunks

-

1 tablespoon vegetable oil

-

1 1/2 cups chopped celery

-

1 1/2 cups chopped carrots

-

6 green onions, chopped

-

1 cup chicken broth

-

1/3 cup soy sauce

-

1/4 teaspoon ground red pepper, or to taste

-

1/2 teaspoon ground ginger

-

1 clove garlic, finely minced

-

1 can (approximately 12 to 15 ounces) ounces bean sprouts, drained

-

1 can (8 ounces) sliced water chestnuts, drained

- 1/4 cup cornstarch

- 1/3 cup water

PREPARATION

1.

In a large skillet, brown chicken pieces. Put browned chicken in the slow cooker. Add remaining ingredients except cornstarch and water. Stir. Cover and cook on LOW for 6 to 8 hours. Turn the slow cooker to HIGH . Mix cornstarch and water in a small bowl, stirring until dissolved and smooth. Stir into the slow cooker liquids. Keeping cover slightly ajar to allow steam to escape, cook until thickened, about 20 to 30 minutes.

2.

Serve with rice or chow mein noodles. May be doubled for 5 qt. slow cooker/Crock Pots.

Crockpot Chicken Cordon Bleu

INGREDIENTS

- 4-6 chicken breasts (pounded out thin)

- 4-6 pieces of ham

- 4-6 slices of Swiss or mozzarella cheese

- 1 can cream of mushroom soup (can use any cream soup)

- 1/4 cup milk

PREPARATION

1.
Put ham and cheese on chicken. Roll up and secure with a toothpick. Place chicken in the slow cooker/Crock Pot so it looks like a triangle /_\ Layer the rest on top. Mix soup with the milk; pour over top of chicken. Cover and cook on low for 4 hours or until chicken is no longer pink. Serve over noodles with the sauce it makes.

2.
Teresa's Note: Its the best recipe I've tried so far, very flavorful.

Crockpot Chicken Cordon Bleu II

INGREDIENTS

- 6 chicken breast halves

- 6 slices ham

- 6 slices Swiss cheese

- 1/2 c. flour

- 1/2 c. Parmesan cheese

- 1/2 tsp. salt

- 1/4 tsp. pepper

- 3 tablespoons oil

- 1 can cream of chicken soup

- 1/2 cup dry white wine

PREPARATION

1.

Place each chicken breast half between pieces of plastic wrap and pound gently to flatten to an even thickness. Place a slice of ham and a slice of Swiss cheese on each chicken breast; roll up and secure with toothpicks or kitchen twine. Combine flour, Parmesan cheese, salt and pepper in bowl. Roll chicken in the Parmesan and flour mixture; chill 1 hour. After chilling the chicken, heat a skillet with 3 tablespoons oil; brown chicken on all sides.

2.

In crockpot combine chicken soup and wine. Add browned chicken and cook on LOW for 4 1/2 to 5 1/2 hours or HIGH for about 2 1/2 hours. Thicken sauce with a mixture of flour and cold water (about 2 tablespoons flour whisked with 2 tablespoons cold water). Cook for about 20 minutes longer, until thickened.

3.

Serves 6.

Crockpot Chicken Drumsticks

INGREDIENTS

- 12 to 16 chicken drumsticks, skin removed

- 1 cup maple syrup

- 1/2 cup soy sauce

- 1 can (14 ounces) whole berry cranberry sauce

- 1 teaspoon Dijon mustard

- 1 tablespoon cornstarch

- 1 tablespoon cold water

- sliced green onions or fresh chopped cilantro, optional

PREPARATION

1.
If you choose to leave the skin on the drumsticks, put the chicken in a large saucepan, cover with water, and bring to a boil over high heat. Boil for about 5 minutes. Parboiling will remove some of the excess fat from the skin.

2.
Remove the chicken, pat dry, and place the drumsticks in the slow cooker.

3.

In a bowl combine the maple syrup, soy sauce, cranberry sauce, and mustard. Pour over the drumsticks.

4.

Cover and cook for 6 to 7 hours on LOW or about 3 hours on HIGH. The chicken should be very tender, but not completely falling apart.

5.

Remove the chicken drumsticks to a platter and keep warm.

6.

Combine the cornstarch and cold water in a cup or small bowl. Stir until smooth.

7.

Increase the slow cooker temperature to high and stir in the cornstarch mixture. Cook for about 10 minutes, until thickened.

8.

Or transfer the liquids to a saucepan and bring to a boil. Stir in the cornstarch mixture and cook, stirring for a minute or two until the sauce has thickened.

9.

Serve garnished with sliced green onions or chopped cilantro if desired.

10.
Variations

11.

Use bone-in chicken thighs or in place of the drumsticks. Remove the skin before cooking.

12.

Use 6 to 8 whole, skinless chicken legs instead of drumsticks.

Crockpot Chicken Fricassee Recipe

INGREDIENTS

- 1 can condensed cream of chicken soup, reduced fat or Healthy Request

- 1/4 cup water

- 1/2 cup chopped onions

- 1 teaspoon ground paprika

- 1 teaspoon lemon juice

- 1 teaspoon dried rosemary, crushed

- 1 teaspoon thyme

- 1 teaspoon parsley flakes

- 1 teaspoon salt

- 1/4 teaspoon pepper

- 4 boneless chicken breast halves, without skin

- non-stick cooking spray

-

Chive Dumplings

-

3 tablespoons shortening

-

1 1/2 cups flour

-

2 tsp. baking powder

-

3/4 tsp. salt

-

3 tablespoons fresh chopped chives or parsley

-

3/4 cup skim milk

PREPARATION

1.
Spray slow cooker with non-stick cooking spray. Place chicken in slow cooker.

2.
Combine soup, water, onions, paprika, lemon juice, rosemary, thyme, parsley, 1 teaspoon salt, and pepper; pour over chicken. Cover and cook on LOW for 6 to 7 hours. One hour before serving time, prepare the dumplings, below.

3.
Dumplings:

4.

With pastry blender or forks, work dry ingredients and shortening together until the mixture resembles coarse meal.

5.

Add chives or parsley and milk; mix just until well combined. With teaspoon, drop onto hot chicken and gravy. Cover and continue cooking on HIGH for about 25 minutes longer, until dumplings are cooked. Serve with mashed potatoes or noodles, along with vegetables or a salad.

Crockpot Chicken Reuben Casserole

INGREDIENTS

-

2 bags (16 ounces each) sauerkraut, rinsed and drained

-

1 cup light or low calorie Russian salad dressing, divided

-

6 boneless chicken breast halves, without skin

-

1 tablespoon prepared mustard

-

4 to 6 slices Swiss cheese

-

fresh parsley, for garnish, optional

PREPARATION

1.

Place half the sauerkraut in a 3 1/2 quart electric slow cooker. Drizzle on about 1/3 cup of the dressing. Top with 3 chicken breast halves and spread the mustard over the chicken. Top with the remaining sauerkraut and chicken breasts. Drizzle another 1/3 cup dressing over the casserole. Refrigerate the remaining dressing until serving them. Cover and cook on the low heat setting about 3 1/2 to 4 hours, or until the chicken is white throughout and tender.

2.

To serve, spoon the casserole onto 6 plates. Top each with a slice of cheese and drizzle with a few teaspoons of the Russian dressing. Serve immediately, garnished with fresh parsley, if desired.

3.

Serves 6.

Crockpot Chicken With Artichokes

INGREDIENTS

- 1 1/2 to 2 pounds boneless chicken breast halves, skin removed

- 8 ounces sliced fresh mushrooms

- 1 can (14.5 ounces) diced tomatoes

- 1 package frozen artichokes, 8 to 12 ounces

- 1 cup chicken broth

- 1/2 cup chopped onion

- 1 can (3 to 4 ounces) sliced ripe olives

- 1/4 cup dry white wine or chicken broth

- 3 tablespoons quick-cooking tapioca

- 2 teaspoons curry powder, or to taste

- 3/4 teaspoon dried thyme, crushed

- 1/4 teaspoon salt

-

1/4 teaspoon pepper

-

4 cups hot cooked rice

PREPARATION

1.

Rinse chicken; pat dry and set aside. In a 3 1/2 to 5-quart slow cooker combine the mushrooms, tomatoes, artichoke hearts, chicken broth, chopped onion, sliced olives, and wine. Stir in tapioca, curry powder, thyme, salt, and pepper. Add chicken to crockpot; spoon some of the tomato mixture over chicken.

2.

Cover and cook on LOW for 7 to 8 hours or on HIGH for 3 1/2 to 4 hours. Serve with hot cooked rice.

3.

Makes 6 to 8 servings.

Crockpot Chicken with Dijon Mustard

INGREDIENTS

- 4 to 6 boneless chicken breast halves

- 2 tablespoons Dijon mustard

- 1 can 98% fat-free cream of mushroom soup

- 2 teaspoons cornstarch

- dash black pepper

PREPARATION

1.
Place the chicken breast halves in the slow cooker insert.

2.
Combine remaining ingredients and spoon over the chicken.

3.
Cover and cook on low 6 to 8 hours.

Crockpot Chicken With Rice

INGREDIENTS

- 4 to 6 boneless chicken breast halves, without skin

- 1 can (10 3/4 ounces) condensed cream of mushroom soup or cream of chicken

- 1/2 cup water

- 3/4 cup converted rice, uncooked

- 1 1/2 cups chicken broth

- 1 to 2 cups frozen green beans, thawed

PREPARATION

1.

Put chicken breasts in the Crock Pot. Add cream of mushroom soup and 1/2 cup water.

2.

Add 3/4 cup of rice and the chicken broth.

3.

Add green beans.

4.

Cover and cook on LOW for 6 hours, or until chicken is cooked and rice is tender.

Serves 4 to 6.

Crockpot Chicken With Tomatoes

INGREDIENTS

-
  4 to 6 chicken breast halves

-
  2 green bell peppers, sliced

-
  1 can chopped stewed tomatoes

-
  1/2 small bottle Italian dressing (low-fat if desired)

PREPARATION

1.
Place chicken breasts, green bell peppers, stewed tomatoes and Italian dressing in the slow cooker or crockpot and cook all day (6 to 8 hours) on low.

2.
This recipe for chicken with stewed tomatoes shared by Myron in Florida

Crockpot Cola Chicken

INGREDIENTS

-
1 whole chicken, about 3 pounds

-
1 cup ketchup

-
1 large onion, thinly sliced

-
1 cup cola, Coke, Pepsi, Dr. Pepper, etc.

PREPARATION

1.
Wash and pat chicken dry. Salt and pepper to taste. Put chicken in Crock Pot with the onions on top. Add cola and ketchup and cook on LOW 6 to 8 hours. Enjoy!

2.
Posted by Molly

Crockpot Creole Chicken

INGREDIENTS

- 1 pound boneless chicken thighs, skin removed, cut into 1-inch pieces

- 1 can (14.5 ounces) tomatoes with juice

- 1 1/2 cups chicken broth

- 8 ounces fully cooked smoked sausage, sliced

- 1/2 to 1 cup diced cooked ham

- 1 cup chopped onion

- 1 can (6 ounces) tomato paste

- 1/4 cup water

- 1 1/2 teaspoons Creole seasoning

- a few dashes of Tabasco sauce or other hot pepper sauce

- 2 cups instant rice, uncooked•

- 1 cup chopped green bell pepper

PREPARATION

1.

Combine chicken, tomatoes, broth, sausage, ham, onion, tomato paste, water, seasoning, and Tabasco sauce in the slow cooker. Cover and cook on LOW for 5 to 6 hours.

2.

Add rice• and green pepper to crockpot and cook for 10 minutes longer, or until rice is tender and most of the liquid is absorbed.

3.

If desired, cook 1 1/2 cups of regular long grain rice and serve along with the chicken mixture.

4.

Serves 6.

Crockpot Herb Chicken With Stuffing

INGREDIENTS

- 1 can (10 1/2 ounces) cream of chicken with herbs soup

- 1 can (10 1/2 ounces) cream of celery or cream of chicken soup

- 1/2 cup dry white wine or chicken broth

- 1 teaspoon dried parsley flakes

- 1 teaspoon dried leaf thyme, crumbled

- 1/2 teaspoon salt

- Dash black pepper

- 2 to 2 1/2 cups seasoned stuffing crumbs, about 6 ounces, divided

- 4 tablespoons butter, divided

- 6 to 8 boneless chicken breast halves, without skin

PREPARATION

1.

2.

Combine the soups, wine or broth, parsley, thyme, salt, and pepper.

3.

Wash chicken and pat dry.

4.

Lightly grease a 5 to 7-quart slow cooker insert.

5.

Sprinkle about 1/2 cup of the stuffing crumbs over the bottom of the cooker and drizzle with about 1 tablespoon of the butter.

6.

Top with half of the chicken, then half of the remaining stuffing crumbs. Drizzle with half of the remaining butter and spoon half of the soup mixture over that.

1.

Repeat with remaining chicken, stuffing crumbs, butter, and soup mixture.

2.

Cover and cook on LOW for 5 to 7 hours, or until chicken is cooked through.

Serves 6 to 8.

Crockpot Herb Chicken With Stuffing

INGREDIENTS

-

1 can (10 1/2 ounces) cream of chicken with herbs soup

-

1 can (10 1/2 ounces) cream of celery or cream of chicken soup

-

1/2 cup dry white wine or chicken broth

-

1 teaspoon dried parsley flakes

-

1 teaspoon dried leaf thyme, crumbled

-

1/2 teaspoon salt

-

Dash black pepper

-

2 to 2 1/2 cups seasoned stuffing crumbs, about 6 ounces, divided

-

4 tablespoons butter, divided

-

6 to 8 boneless chicken breast halves, without skin

PREPARATION

1.

Combine the soups, wine or broth, parsley, thyme, salt, and pepper.

2.

Wash chicken and pat dry.

3.

Lightly grease a 5 to 7-quart slow cooker insert.

4.

Sprinkle about 1/2 cup of the stuffing crumbs over the bottom of the cooker and drizzle with about 1 tablespoon of the butter.

5.

Top with half of the chicken, then half of the remaining stuffing crumbs. Drizzle with half of the remaining butter and spoon half of the soup mixture over that.

1.

Repeat with remaining chicken, stuffing crumbs, butter, and soup mixture.

2.

Cover and cook on LOW for 5 to 7 hours, or until chicken is cooked through.

Serves 6 to 8.

Crockpot Italian-Style Chicken

INGREDIENTS

- 4 pounds chicken pieces

- 3 tablespoons olive oil

- 2 onions, sliced

- 1 teaspoon salt

- 1/2 teaspoon fresh ground pepper

- 2 celery ribs, cut in small chunks

- 2 cups diced potatoes

- 1 can (14.5 ounces) diced tomatoes, undrained

- 1 teaspoon dried leaf oregano

- 1 tablespoon dried parsley flakes

- 1 cup frozen peas, thawed

PREPARATION

1.

Brown the chicken parts in hot oil. Add salt, pepper and onions and cook for another 5 minutes. Put celery and potatoes in the bottom of the slow cooker and top with browned chicken, onions, and tomatoes with juice, oregano, and parsley. Cover and cook on low for 6 to 8 hours. Add peas the last 30 minutes.

2.

Serves 6.

Crock Pot Lima Beans with Chicken

INGREDIENTS

- 3 to 4 pounds chicken pieces

- salt and pepper

- 1 tablespoon vegetable oil

- 2 large potatoes, cut in 1-inch cubes

- 1 package frozen lima beans, thawed

- 1 cup chicken broth

- 1/4 teaspoon dried leaf thyme, crumbled

PREPARATION

1.

Season chicken with salt and pepper. Heat oil and butter in large skillet; fry chicken until browned on both sides. Place chicken in crockpot with remaining ingredients. Cover and cook on low for 4 to 6 hours, until chicken is tender.

2.

Serves 4.

Crockpot Pasta and Cheese Delight

INGREDIENTS

- 1 jar Alfredo Sauce

- 1 can Healthy Request Cream of Mushroom Soup

- 1 (7 oz) can white tuna or chicken, drained, or use leftover cooked chicken or meat

- 1/4 teaspoon curry powder

- 1 to 1 1/2 cups frozen mixed vegetables

- 1 1/2 cups shredded Swiss cheese

- 4 cups cooked pasta (macaroni, bow ties, shells)

PREPARATION

1.

Combine first 5 ingredients; cover and cook for 4 to 5 hours on LOW. Add Swiss cheese to the mixture during the last hour. Cook pasta according to package directions; drain and add to slow cooker. This would be just as good with cooked or canned chicken, leftover ham or just add extra veggies!

2.

Serves 4.

Debbie's Crockpot Chicken and Stuffing

INGREDIENTS

-
1 package herb-seasoned stuffing mix, prepared

-
4 to 6 boneless chicken breast halves or boneless thighs, without skin•

-
1 can (10 3/4 ounces) condensed cream of chicken soup, undiluted

-
1 can (3 to 4 ounces or more) sliced mushrooms, drained

PREPARATION

1.
Butter the bottom and sides of the slow cooker crockery insert.

2.
Prepare the packaged (or homemade) stuffing mix with butter and liquid as directed on package.

3.
Layer the prepared stuffing in the bottom of the greased slow cooker.

4.
Place the chicken pieces on top of the stuffing mixture. The chicken can overlap some, but try to arrange with as little overlap as possible. If there is room, you could use more chicken.

5.
Spoon the condensed cream of chicken soup over the chicken. You may also use cream of mushroom, or cream of celery, whatever you like. Top with the mushrooms. Be sure to stir the mushrooms around a little so they are coated with the soup.

6.

Cover and cook on low for 5 to 7 hours.

7.

•Chicken breasts tend to become dry over a long period of cooking, so check them early. Thighs are fattier than the chicken breasts, so they can be cooked for a longer period of time.

Diana's Chicken a la King

INGREDIENTS

- 1 1/2 to 2 pounds boneless chicken tenders

- 1 to 1 1/2 cup matchstick-cut carrots

- 1 bunch green onions (scallions) sliced in 1/2-inch pieces

- 1 jar Kraft pimiento or pimiento & olive process cheese spread (5oz)

- 1 can 98% fat-free cream of chicken soup

- 2 tablespoons dry sherry (optional)

- salt and pepper to taste

PREPARATION

1.
Put all ingredients in the slow cooker/Crock Pot (3 1/2-quart or larger) in the order given; stir to combine. Cover and cook on low for 7 to 9 hours. Serve over rice, toast, or biscuits.

2.
Serves 6 to 8.

Dilled Chicken with Veggies

INGREDIENTS

- 1 to 1 1/2 pounds chicken tenders, cut in 1-inch pieces

- 1 tablespoon dried minced onion (or small onion, chopped)

- 1 can regular or 98% fat reduced cream of mushroom soup

- 1 packet (1oz) mushroom gravy mix (chicken or country gravy may be substituted)

- 1 cup baby carrots

- 1/2 to 1 teaspoon dill weed

- seasoned salt and pepper to taste

- 1 cup frozen peas

PREPARATION

1.
Combine first 7 ingredients in the slow cooker/Crock Pot; cover and cook on low for 6 to 8 hours. Add frozen peas during the last 30 to 45 minutes. Serve with rice or mashed potatoes.

2.
Serves 4.

Don's Sweet and Sour Chicken

INGREDIENTS

- 2 to 4 skinless chicken breasts

- 1 large onion roughly chopped

- 2 bell peppers roughly chopped (one green, one red)

- 1 cup of broccoli florettes

- 1/2 cup of carrot chunks

- 1 large can of chunk pineapple (drain and SAVE the juice)

- 1/4-1/2 cup of brown sugar(can use reg. sugar)

- Water/wine/white grape juice/orange juice etc. as needed for extra liquid

- 1 Tablespoon of cornstarch for every cup of liquid you end up with

- hot sauce to taste, optional

- salt and pepper to taste, optional

- cinnamon, optional

-

allspice, optional

-

cloves, optional

-

curry powder, optional

PREPARATION

1.

Put chicken breasts in slow cooker or crockpot. Add the onion, peppers, broccoli, and carrots Whisk together until blended well, no lumps in sugar, liquids, spices, and cornstarch, and sugar. Pour over chicken. If there is not enough juice, add whichever liquid you prefer to bring up to the desired level. (REMEMBER THOUGH: For each extra cup of liquid, stir in another Tablespoon of cornstarch before you pour it in the slow cooker) .

2.

Cover and cook 6 to 8 hours on LOW. I sometimes vary the recipe, using fruit cocktail and a bit less sugar, pineapple, or apricot preserves or orange marmalade works too. (no cornstarch needed when you used preserves, nor sugar of course. Use your imagination. Remember sweet and sour is basically a fruit juice and vinegar.

Easy Cheesy Slow Cooker Chicken

INGREDIENTS

- 6 boneless chicken breast halves, without skin

- salt and pepper, to taste

- garlic powder, to taste

- 2 cans condensed cream of chicken soup

- 1 can condensed cheddar cheese soup

PREPARATION

1.
Rinse chicken and sprinkle with salt, pepper and garlic powder. Mix undiluted soup and pour over chicken in a Crock Pot.

2.
Cover and cook on low 6 to 8 hours.

3.
Serve over rice or noodles.

4.
Serves 6.

Easy Chicken Cacciatore

INGREDIENTS

- 1 chicken, cut up, about 3 to 3 1/2 pounds

- 1 jar spaghetti sauce

- chopped onions

- sliced mushrooms

- chopped green pepper

- salt and pepper

- red pepper flakes

PREPARATION

1.
Place a whole cut-up chicken (3 to 3 1/2 pounds) in the slow cooker/Crock Pot. Dump in a jar of spaghetti sauce, some cut up onions, mushrooms and green peppers. Salt and pepper to taste. (I use those little red pepper flakes too.)

2.
Cook all day on low (7 to 9 hours). Serve over noodles or spaghetti.

Easy Chicken Pasta Sauce

INGREDIENTS

- 1 lb chicken tenders or chicken breasts, cubed

- 1 can (15 oz) tomatoes, diced

- 1 small can (6 oz) tomato paste

- 1 rib celery, sliced

- 1/4 cup chopped onion

- 1/2 cup chopped or shredded carrots, canned or cooked until slightly tender

- 1/2 tsp oregano

- 1/2 tsp salt

- 1/4 tsp pepper

- 1/2 tsp garlic powder

- pinch of sugar or other sweetener (optional or to taste)

PREPARATION

1.

Combine all ingredients in slow cooker or crockpot. Cover and cook on low for 6 to 8 hours. Taste and adjust seasonings about 30 minutes before serving and add a little water to thin, if necessary. Serve this easy recipe for chicken pasta sauce over spaghetti, fettucine or other pasta.

2.

This easy recipe with chicken serves 4.

Easy Chicken With Almonds

INGREDIENTS

- 4 to 6 chicken breast halves, washed, skin removed

- 1 can (10 3/4 oz) cream of chicken soup

- 1 tablespoon lemon juice

- 1/3 cup mayonnaise

- 1/2 cup thinly sliced celery

- 1/4 cup finely chopped onions

- 1/4 cup drained chopped pimiento

- 1/2 cup slivered or sliced almonds

- chopped fresh parsley, optional

PREPARATION

1.
Arrange chicken breasts in the bottom of the slow cooker. In a bowl combine soup, lemon juice, mayonnaise, celery, onions, and pimiento; pour over chicken breasts. Cover and cook on low 5 to 7 hours, until chicken is tender (boneless chicken breast halves will take less time than bone-in). Remove chicken breasts to a serving plate and spoon juices over them. Top with a sprinkling of almonds and parsley, if desired.

2.
Serve with hot cooked rice and steamed broccoli.

3.
Serves 4 to 6.

Easy Crockpot Cassoulet

INGREDIENTS

-

1 tablespoon extra virgin olive oil

-

1 large onion, finely chopped

-

4 boneless skinless chicken thighs, coarsely chopped

-

1/4 pound cooked smoked sausage, such as kielbasa or spicier andouille, diced

-

3 cloves garlic, minced

-

1 teaspoon dried thyme leaves

-

1/2 teaspoon black pepper

-

4 tablespoons tomato paste

-

2 tablespoons water

-

3 cans (about 15 ounces each) great northern beans, rinsed and drained

-

3 tablespoons chopped fresh parsley

PREPARATION

1.

Heat olive oil in large skillet over medium heat.

2.

Add onion to hot oil and cook, stirring, until onion is tender, about 4 minutes.

3.

Stir in chicken, sausage, garlic, thyme, and pepper. Cook 5 to 8 minutes, or until chicken and sausage are browned.

4.

Stir in tomato paste and water; transfer to slow cooker. Stir great northern beans into the chicken mixture; cover and cook on LOW for 4 to 6 hours.

5.

Before serving, sprinkle the chopped parsley over cassoulet.

6.

Serves 6.

Easy Crockpot Chicken Santa Fe From Cindy

INGREDIENTS

- 1 can (15 oz) black beans, rinsed and drained

- 2 cans (15 oz) whole kernel corn, drained

- 1 cup bottled thick and chunky salsa, your favorite

- 5 or 6 skinless, boneless chicken breast halves (about 2 lbs)

- 1 cup shredded Cheddar cheese

PREPARATION

1.
In a 3-1/2- to 5-quart slow cooker, mix together the black beans, corn, and 1/2 cup of the salsa.

2.
Top with the chicken breasts, then pour the remaining 1/2 cup salsa over the chicken. Cover and cook on HIGH for 2 1/2 to 3 hours, or until the chicken is tender and white throughout. Do not overcook or the chicken will be dry.

3.
Sprinkle cheese on top; cover and cook until the cheese melts, about 5 to 15 minutes.

4.
Serves 6.

Seafood Crockpot

INGREDIENTS

- 2 cans shrimp (approx. 5 ounces each), drain

- 2 cans tuna (approx. 7 ounces each), flaked

- 2 cans crabmeat (approx. 7 ounces each), pick over, remove cartilage

- 1 can chopped pimiento (4 ounces), drained

- 1/3 cup minced fresh parsley

- 3 cups instant rice, uncooked

- 2 cans condensed cream of mushroom soup

- 3 cups water

- 1/2 cup dry white wine

- 1/4 cup onion, chopped

- 2 teaspoons dill weed

- 1/2 teaspoon paprika

- 1/2 teaspoon Tabasco sauce

PREPARATION

1. Place first six ingredients in crockpot. Combine cream of mushroom soup with water, wine, onion, dillweed, paprika and Tabasco sauce. Pour over rice and seafood mixture in crockpot; stir gently to blend well.
2. Cover and cook on low for 3 to 4 hours, until rice is tender.

Salmon and Potato Casserole

INGREDIENTS

- 4 to 5 medium potatoes, peeled and sliced

- 3 tablespoons flour

- salt and pepper

- 1 can (16 ounces) salmon, drained and flaked

- 1/2 cup chopped onion

- 1 can (10 3/4 ounces) cream of mushroom soup or cream of celery soup

- 1/4 cup water

- dash nutmeg

PREPARATION

1. Place half of the potatoes in greased slow cooker/Crock Pot. Sprinkle with half of the flour, then sprinkle lightly with salt and pepper. Cover with half the flaked salmon; sprinkle with half the onion. Repeat layers. Combine soup and water; pour over top of potato and salmon mixture. Sprinkle with just a dash of nutmeg. Cover and cook on Low for 7 to 9 hours, or until potatoes are tender.
2. Serves 6.

Shrimp Creole

INGREDIENTS

- 1 1/2 cups diced celery

- 1 1/4 cups chopped onion

- 1 cup chopped bell pepper

- 1 (8 oz.) can tomato sauce

- 1 (28 oz.) can whole tomatoes, broken up

- 1 clove garlic, minced

- 1 teaspoon salt, or to taste

- 1/2 teaspoon Creole seasoning

- 1/4 teaspoon freshly ground black pepper

- 6 drops Tabasco, or to taste

- 1 to 1 1/2 pounds shrimp, deveined & shelled

PREPARATION

1. Combine all ingredients except shrimp. Cook 3 to 4 hours on high or 6 to 8 hours on low. Add shrimp last hour of cooking. Serve over hot rice. Chicken, rabbit or crawfish may be substituted for shrimp. Stove top version, if you don't have a Crock Pot. Saute celery, onion and bell peppers in oil or butter until tender. Add remaining ingredients except shrimp. Simmer at least 30 minutes to an hour. Add shrimp (or cubed cooked chicken or other seafood) and simmer 30 minutes more.
2. This is even better reheated the next day.

Sweet and Sour Shrimp

INGREDIENTS

-

1 package (6 ounces) frozen Chinese pea pods

-

1 can (12 to 14 ounces) pineapple tidbits in juice

-

2 tablespoons cornstarch

-

3 tablespoons granulated sugar

-

1 cup chicken broth

-

1/2 cup reserved pineapple juice

-

1 tablespoon soy sauce

-

1/2 tsp ground ginger

-

1 bag (12 to 16 ounces) frozen small to medium shrimp, cleaned and cooked

-

2 tablespoons cider vinegar

-

hot cooked rice

PREPARATION

1. Put pea pods in a colander and run cold water over them until partially thawed -- enough to separate easily. Drain pineapple, reserving 1/2 cup of the juice. Place pea pods and drained pineapple in slow cooker. In a small saucepan, stir together cornstarch and sugar; add chicken broth, reserved pineapple juice, soy sauce, and ginger. Bring mixture to a boil, stirring, and cook sauce for about 1 minute.

2. The sauce should be thickened and clear. Gently blend sauce into pea pods and pineapple. Cover and cook on LOW for 3 to 5 hours. Add the thawed cooked shrimp; continue to cook 30 minutes longer, until heated through. Add vinegar and stir gently.

3. Serve with hot cooked rice.

Tuna Noodle Casserole

INGREDIENTS

- 1/4 cup dry sherry

- 2/3 cup Milk

- 2 tablespoons parsley flakes

- 10 ounces frozen peas and carrots, about 1 1/2 to 2 cups

- 2 cans tuna, drained

- 1/4 teaspoon curry powder, or to taste

- 10 ounces egg noodles, cooked until just tender

- 2 tablespoons butter

PREPARATION

1. In a large mixing bowl, cream of celery combine soup, sherry, milk, parsley flakes, vegetables, curry powder, and tuna. Fold in noodles; mix to combine well. Pour mixture into a generously greased slow cooker. Dot with butter. Cover and cook on Low 5 to 7 hours, until vegetables are done and noodles are tender.

Tuna Noodle Casserole #2

INGREDIENTS

- 2 cans cream of celery soup

- 1/3 cup chicken broth

- 2/3 cup milk

- 2 tablespoons dried parsley flakes

- 1 package (10 ounces) frozen peas, thawed

- 2 (7 ounces each) cans tuna, drained

- 10 ounces medium egg noodles, cooked until just tender

- 3 tablespoons buttered bread crumbs or potato chip crumbs

PREPARATION

1. Grease bottom and sides of the slow cooker insert (a 4 to 5-quart crockpot). In a large bowl, combine soup, chicken broth, milk, parsley, vegetables, and tuna. Fold in the cooked noodles. Pour mixture into prepared slow cooker. Top with buttered bread crumbs or potato chip crumbs. Cover and cook on LOW for 5 to 6 hours. Serves 4 to 6.

Tuna Salad Casserole

INGREDIENTS

- 2 cans tuna, drained and flaked

- 1 can cream of celery soup

- 4 hard-cooked eggs, chopped

- 1 cup diced celery

- 1/2 cup mayonnaise

- 1/4 tsp. pepper

- 1 1/2 cups crushed potato chips

PREPARATION

1. Grease slow cooker or spray with non-stick cooking spray. Combine all ingredients except 1/4 cup of the crushed potato chips; stir well. Pour into prepared slow cooker.
2. Top with remaining potato chips.
3. Cover and cook on LOW for 4 to 6 hours.

White Beans and Tomatoes With Tuna

INGREDIENTS

- 4 tablespoons olive oil

- 1 clove garlic, crushed

- 1 pound small white beans, soaked overnight drained

- 2 cups chopped tomatoes

- 2 6-1/2oz can white tuna in water, drained and flaked

- 2 sprigs basil, finely chopped, or 1 1/2 teaspoons dried basil

- salt and pepper, to taste

PREPARATION

1. Saute garlic in oil until brown; discard garlic. Combine the garlic flavored oil with beans and 6 cups water (48 ounces) in crockpot. Cover and cook on high 2 hours. Turn heat to low, cover and cook 8 hours. Add remaining ingredients; cover and cook on high for 30 minutes.

Will's Crockpot Cioppino

INGREDIENTS

- 1 large can (28 ounces) crushed tomatoes with juice

- 1 can (8 ounces) tomato sauce

- 1/2 cup chopped onion

- 1 cup dry white wine

- 1/3 cup olive oil

- 3 cloves garlic, minced

- 1/2 cup parsley, chopped

- 1 green pepper, chopped

- 1 hot pepper (optional), chopped

- salt and pepper, to taste

- 1 teaspoon thyme

- 2 teaspoons basil

-

1 teaspoon oregano

-

1/2 teaspoon paprika

-

1/2 teaspoon cayenne pepper

-

water, if desired•

-

Seafood••

-

1 deboned (important) and cubed fillet of seabass, cod or other whitefish

-

1 doz. prawns

-

1 doz. scallops

-

1 doz. mussels

-

1 doz. clams (can use canned)

PREPARATION

1. Place all ingredients in slow cooker except seafood. Cover and cook 6 to 8 hours on low.
2. About 30 minutes before serving, add your seafood. Turn the heat up to HIGH and stir occasionally (but gently).
3. Serve with true sourdough bread if you can find it. We here in San Francisco are lucky in that we have a choice of several

really 'sour' tasting brands. By the way, don't be afraid to dunk your bread in the chioppino as it's considered perfectly good manners in this case.

Will's Notes:

•You can add water to the recipe to thin out the Cioppino somewhat but we prefer it nice and thick.

••Use your imagination and personal preferences as to which seafoods to add. Some choose to serve with fresh cracked crab when in season.

Apple-Apricot Chops

INGREDIENTS

- 2 pounds pork filets or chops

- 1 cup chopped apple

- 1 cup chopped dried apricot

- 1 medium onion, chopped

- 2 ribs celery, sliced in 1/2-inch pieces

- 1/2 cup apple juice

- 1/2 cup brown sugar

- 1/4 cup dry sherry or dry white wine, or more apple juice

- salt and pepper to taste

- 1 1/2 tablespoons cornstarch mixed with 2 tablespoons cold water

PREPARATION

1. Combine all ingredients; cover and cook on LOW for 7 to 9 hours, or 3 1/2 to 4 1/2 hours on HIGH. About 20 to 30 minutes before serving, pour liquid into a separate container to skim off excess fat. Stir in cornstarch mixture and return broth to slow cooker. Continue cooking on low until sauce is smooth and thickened.
2. Serves 4 to 6.

Apple-icious Pork Tenderloins

INGREDIENTS

- 2 pork tenderloins (1 1/2 to 2 lbs total)

- 1 large onion, halved and cut in 1/4-inch slices

- 2 apples, peeled and coarsely chopped

- 2 tablespoons apple jelly

- 1 tablespoon cider vinegar

- salt and coarsely ground black pepper to taste

PREPARATION

1. Combine all ingredients in the slow cooker/Crock Pot (brown pork if desired). Cover and cook on low for 7 to 9 hours. Serve with rice.
2. Serves 4 to 6.

Apple Sausage With Onion and Mustard Sauce

INGREDIENTS

- 1 1/2 to 2 pounds chicken apple sausage links or similar smoked sausage

- 1 medium sweet onion, sliced

- 4 tablespoons Creole mustard or other grainy mustard

- 4 tablespoons balsamic vinegar

- 4 tablespoons brown sugar

- 3 tablespoons honey

PREPARATION

1. Cut sausages into 1- to 2-inch chunks. Put sliced onion in the bottom of a slow cooker; top with the sliced sausages. Combine remaining ingredients in a large cup or small bowl and pour over the sausages. Cover and cook on LOW for 5 to 7 hours, or on HIGH for 2 1/2 to 3 1/2 hours. Serve with rice or noodles and a side vegetable, or cut into smaller pieces and serve as an appetizer. Serves 6 to 8 as a main dish.

Auntie's Bar-B-Q

INGREDIENTS

-

1 1/2 pounds lean beef, cut in 1 to 2-inch cubes

-

1 1/2 pounds pork, cut in 1 to 2-inch cubes

-

2 cups chopped onion

-

1/4 cup chopped green pepper

-

1 (6 oz.) can tomato paste

-

1/2 cup brown sugar

-

1/4 cup vinegar

-

1 tsp. salt

-

2 tsp. Worcestershire sauce

-

1 tsp. dry mustard

PREPARATION

1. Combine all ingredients in slow cooker. Cover and cook on LOW for 9 to 11 hours, until very tender, or on HIGH for 5 to 6 hours. Stir, breaking up meat, and serve with warm split sandwich rolls.
2. Serves 8.

Autumn Pork Roast

INGREDIENTS

- pork loin roast, 3 to 4 pounds

- salt and pepper

- 1 cup fresh or frozen cranberries, chopped

- 1/4 c. honey

- 1 tsp. grated orange peel

- 1/8 tsp. ground nutmeg

- 1/8 tsp. ground allspice

PREPARATION

1. Sprinkle pork loin roast with salt and pepper. Place in slow cooker or Crock Pot. Combine remaining ingredients and spoon over roast.
2. Cover and cook on LOW for 8 to 10 hours. Makes 6 to 8 servings.

Baby Lima Beans With HamBar-B-Q Pork

INGREDIENTS

- 1 pound dried baby lima beans

- 2 quarts water for soaking

- 2 medium onions, coarsely chopped

- 1 meaty ham bone plus leftover diced ham, as desired

- 3 to 4 cups water, to cover

- 1 teaspoon Cajun or Creole seasoning blend

- 1/4 teaspoon freshly ground black pepper

- dash cayenne pepper

- salt, to taste

PREPARATION

1. Soak the lima beans in about 2 quarts of water overnight.
2. Drain and put lima beans in the slow cooker insert. Add 3 to 4 cups of fresh water just to cover the beans and stir in the chopped onions and add the ham bone and ham.
3. Cover and cook on HIGH for 3 hours.
4. Add the Creole seasoning, and black and cayenne peppers. Cover and cook on LOW for 4 hours, or until very tender.
5.

Serves 8.

Barbeque Pork For Sandwiches

INGREDIENTS

- 3 pounds cubed pork shoulder, or use about half stewing beef

- 1 large onion, chopped

- 1 tsp. salt

- 1 tbsp. chili powder

- 1 chopped green pepper

- 1 cup water

- 2 cups barbecue sauce, divided

- toasted split buns

PREPARATION

1. Put the pork in a slow cooker with the onion, salt, chili powder, bell pepper, and water. Cover and cook on LOW for 7 to 9 hours, or until very tender. Drain and discard excess liquids. Chop or shred the meat and return to the crock pot with 1 cup of the barbecue sauce.
2. Cover and cook on LOW for 1 hour longer. Serve on toasted split buns with the remaining barbecue sauce.

Barbecue Pork Roast

INGREDIENTS

- 1 pork roast, shoulder, butt

- 2 to 3 tablespoons lemon juice

- 1/2 cup coarsely chopped onion

- 1 teaspoon granulated sugar

- 1 bottle barbecue sauce, about 18 ounces

PREPARATION

1. Cook pork roast covered in water (start with hot water) in Crock Pot on low 9 to 11 hours, or until very tender and falling apart. Pour off water and shred meat; discard fat and bone.
2. Saute onion in a little butter.
3. Combine barbecue sauce, onions, sugar and juice of lemon with meat in Crock Pot and cook on high for about 1 hour, or on low for about 2 hours.
4. Serve shredded pork on buns.
5. Serves 8 to 10, depending on the size of the shoulder.

Barbecued Country Style Ribs

INGREDIENTS

- 3 pounds boneless country-style pork ribs

- 2 large tart apples, peeled, cored, chopped or thinly sliced

- 1 large onion, halved and thinly sliced

- 1/4 teaspoon cinnamon

- Scant 1/4 teaspoon allspice

- salt and pepper

- 1 cup barbecue sauce

PREPARATION

1. In a slow cooker, combine the ribs, apples, onion, cinnamon, and allspice. Sprinkle with salt and pepper.
2. Cover and cook on LOW for 7 to 9 hours. Drain off and discard juices. Add barbecue sauce and continue cooking for about 30 minutes longer.
3. Serves 4 to 6.

BBQ Boston Butt

INGREDIENTS

- pork shoulder or Boston butt, about 4 to 7 pounds, bone-in or boneless

- 1/4 cup of water

- salt and pepper lightly

- barbecue sauce

PREPARATION

1. Place the meat in the slow cooker with water, salt and pepper.
2. Cover and cook on HIGH for 1 hour. Turn to LOW and cook 7 to 9 hours longer, until very tender. Remove roast and discard fat and juices. Chop or shred the pork; return to slow cooker. Mix a little barbecue sauce into the meat for flavor. Cover and cook on LOW for about 1 hour longer, until hot.
3. Serve on warm split sandwich buns with coleslaw and extra barbecue sauce on the side.

Beans and Hot Dogs

INGREDIENTS

- 3 cans (16 ounces each) pork and beans

- 1 pound hot dogs, cut into 1-inch pieces

- 1/2 cup ketchup

- 1 small onion, chopped

- 1/4 cup molasses

- 1 tablespoon prepared mustard

PREPARATION

1. In crockpot, combine beans, hot dogs, ketchup, onion, molasses, and mustard.
2. Cover and cook on LOW for 6 to 8 hours.
3. Serves 6.

Bigos

INGREDIENTS

- 1 can condensed cream of celery soup, undiluted

- 1/3 cup light brown sugar, packed

- 1 can or bag (24 to 32 ounces) sauerkraut, drained and rinsed

- 1 1/2 pounds Polish sausage, cut in 2-inch pieces

- 4 medium potatoes, peeled and cubed

- 1 cup chopped onion

- 1 cup shredded mild Cheddar or Jack cheese

PREPARATION

1. In crockpot, combine the soup, sugar, and sauerkraut. Stir in sausage, potato, and onion. Cover and cook on LOW for 8 hours. Skim off excess fat; stir in cheese. Spoon into serving bowls and top with additional shredded cheese.
2. Serves 6.

Blackbird's Pork Chops

INGREDIENTS

- 6 to 8 Pork Chops

- 1/2 cup Flour

- 1 tbsp salt

- 1 1/2 tsp Dry Mustard

- 1/2 tsp Garlic Powder

- 2 tbsp Oil

- 1 can Chicken and Rice soup

PREPARATION

1. Mix flour, salt, mustard, garlic powder. Dredge chops and brown in oil on stovetop. When browned, place in crock and top with soup. Cover and cook for 6 to 8 hours LOW or about 3 1/2 hours on HIGH.
2. Pork chop recipe shared on our forum by Blackbird.

Crockpot Black Eyed Peas and Ham

INGREDIENTS

-
1 pound frozen black eyed peas

-
1 cup chicken broth

-
2 ribs celery, thinly sliced

-
4 cloves garlic, minced

-
1 bunch (6 to 8) green onions, thinly sliced

-
6 ounces diced ham

-
1/8 teaspoon coarsely ground black pepper

-
1/2 teaspoon Creole seasoning

PREPARATION

1. Combine all ingredients in slow cooker. Cover and cook on LOW for 6 to 8 hours.
2. Serves 6.

Braised Pork Chops

INGREDIENTS

-

6 to 8 lean pork chops

-

1/3 c. flour

-

1 tsp. salt

-

1 tsp. dry mustard

-

1 tablespoon oil

-

1 medium onion, chopped

-

1 large clove garlic minced (optional)

-

1 can cream of chicken soup

PREPARATION

1. Coat chops with mixture of flour, salt, mustard, and garlic salt. Brown on both sides in hot oil in skillet with chopped onion. Add garlic for the last minute. Deglaze the pan with a little water, wine, or broth. Put chops in slow cooker and add soup and pan drippings. Cover and cook on low 6 to 8 hours, or on high 3 to 4 hours.
2. Serves 6 to 8.

Braised Pork Loin

INGREDIENTS

- 3 to 4 pound boneless pork loin roast, trimmed

- 4 cloves garlic, sliced

- salt and pepper

- 1/2 teaspoon each sage and thyme, or 1 teaspoon poultry seasoning

- 1 cup chicken broth

- 1/4 cup dry white wine or chicken broth

- 1/4 cup flour

PREPARATION

1. Brown pork roast on all sides in a large skillet to remove excess fat. Make cuts in roast with a small knife and insert garlic slices; place in slow cooker and season with salt, pepper, and sage and thyme or poultry seasoning. Add broth and wine, if used.
2. Cover and cook on LOW for 8 to 10 hours. Remove roast and skim excess fat from juices; combine flour with about 3 tablespoons cold water and whisk until smooth.
3. Turn the slow cooker to high and stir in the flour mixture. Cook and stir until thickened (this can be done more quickly on the stovetop).
4. Serve sauce over pork, with rice or potatoes.
5. Serves about 8.

Brown Sugar Pork Loin

INGREDIENTS

- 1 boneless pork loin roast, 4 to 6 pounds

- 1 clove garlic, halved

- salt and freshly ground black pepper

- 1 1/3 cups brown sugar, divided

- 1 tablespoon Dijon mustard or a grainy mustard

- 1 tablespoon balsamic vinegar

- 1/4 teaspoon cinnamon

PREPARATION

1. If the pork has an excessive layer of fat, trim it a bit. A little fat will help keep the roast juicy over the long period of cooking.
2. Rub the roast all over with the garlic halves, then sprinkle with salt and pepper, then prick the roast all over with a fork or skewer.
3. In a cup or bowl, combine 1 cup of the brown sugar, the mustard, and vinegar. Rub all over the roast.
4. Cover and cook on LOW for 7 to 9 hours, or until tender but not falling apart.
5. Pour off the excess juices.
6. Combine the remaining 1/3 cup brown sugar with cinnamon; Spread the mixture over the top of the roast. Cover and continue cooking on LOW for 1 hour longer.
7. Serves 6 to 8.

Butterfly Chops & Potatoes

INGREDIENTS

- 6 or more medium red potatoes, thickly sliced

- 1 large onion, quartered and thickly sliced

- 4 to 6 boneless, butterflied pork chops

- 1 packet Zesty Italian dressing mix (0.6oz)

- salt and pepper to taste

PREPARATION

1. Toss potatoes and onion with salt and pepper; top with pork chops. Sprinkle chops with dressing mix. Cover and cook on low 7 to 9 hours. (a 4 1/2-quart or larger pot will be necessary for the larger number of chops & potatoes.)
2. Serves 4 to 6.

Cabbage and Bratwurst

INGREDIENTS

- 5 to 6 links bratwurst sausage

- 1 medium head cabbage, coarsely shredded

- 1 large onion

- 1/2 cup creamy honey-mustard dressing

- 1/4 cup applesauce or apple cider

- 1 to 2 teaspoons caraway seed

- 1/2 teaspoon celery seed

- salt and pepper to taste

PREPARATION

1. Brown sausage and cut into bite-size pieces. Drain well.
2. Combine the browned sausage with cabbage and onion in the Crock Pot.
3. Add remaining ingredients; cover and cook on low for 8 to 10 hours.
4. Serves 4.

Cassoulet with Pork and Beans

INGREDIENTS

- 1 pound cooked navy beans

- 1 bay leaf

- 2 cloves garlic

- 1/2 tsp thyme

- 1/2 tsp sage

- 1 pound lean pork, cubed (chops, cutlets, etc.)

- 1 pound sweet or hot Italian sausages

- 1 cup chicken stock

- Salt and pepper

PREPARATION

1. Place beans in crock with bay, sage, thyme, garlic and seasoning. Fry pork and sausages in frying pan until browned; slice sausages. Add to beans. Add chicken stock and cook on LOW for 7 to 8 hours. If desired, top with buttered bread crumbs and broil until browned.

Catalina Ribs

INGREDIENTS

- 1 1/2 to 2 pounds boneless country style pork ribs

- 1 bottle (8oz) Catalina dressing

- 1 cup chopped onion

- 2 medium cloves garlic, minced

PREPARATION

1. Combine all ingredients in the slow cooker/Crock Pot; cover and cook on low for 7 to 9 hours.
2. Serves 4 to 6.

Chalupas

INGREDIENTS

-

3 to 4 pounds boneless pork loin roast, trimmed

-

2 garlic cloves, minced

-

2 tablespoon chili powder

-

1 tablespoon ground cumin

-

1 teaspoon oregano

-

1 can green chile peppers, chopped

-

2 teaspoons salt, or to taste

-

2 cans (15 ounces each) pinto beans, rinsed and drained

-

••••

-

Suggested Toppings

-

Grated cheese

-

Chopped onions

-

Tomatoes

-

Lettuce

-

Sour cream

-

crushed tortilla chips

PREPARATION

1. Place first 7 ingredients in slow cooker, along with 1/2 cup water. Cook 8 to 10 hours. Add beans 1 hour before done. Top with desired toppings and serve with warm tortillas.

Cherry Pork Chops In Crock Pot

INGREDIENTS

- 6 pork chops, cut 3/4-inch thick

- Salt

- Pepper

- 1 (21 oz.) can cherry pie filling

- 2 tsp. lemon juice

- 1/2 tsp. instant chicken bouillon granules

- 1/8 tsp. ground mace or nutmeg

PREPARATION

1. Brown pork chops quickly in a little fat in a heavy skillet. Sprinkle with salt and pepper. In slow cooker stir together half of the can of cherry pie filling, lemon juice, mace, and bouillon granules. Mix well. Place pork chops on top of mixture. Cover and cook on LOW for 6 to 7 hours. Warm the other half of cherry pie filling and pass in sauce dish when serving chops.
2. Serves 6.

Cherry Glazed Pork Roast

INGREDIENTS

- 1 pork loin roast, boneless, about 3 pounds

- 1 can (10 1/2 ounces) condensed chicken broth

- 1 bunch green onions, with green, sliced in 1-inch lengths

- 3 tablespoons wine vinegar

- 1 teaspoon dried rosemary

- 1/4 teaspoon seasoned pepper (or use regular ground black pepper)

- 1 cup cherry jam, or use apricot or pineapple preserves

- drop or 2 of red food coloring, optional

PREPARATION

1. Trim pork roast and place in slow cooker. Mix all ingredients except jam or preserves and food coloring in small bowl. Pour over roast. Cover and cook on low 8 to 10 hours. Just before serving, turn slow cooker to HIGH.
2. Remove roast to warm serving platter. Mix cherry jam with juices in slow cooker and a little red food coloring, if desired; heat to serving temperature. Spoon over sliced pork.
3. Serves 8.

Chicken-Fried Chops

INGREDIENTS

- 1/2 cup all-purpose flour

- 1 1/2 teaspoons salt

- 1 teaspoon dry mustard

- 1/2 teaspoon paprika

- 1/2 teaspoon garlic powder

- 6 pork loin chops (about 3/4 inch thick) trimmed

- 2 tablespoons canola oil

- 1 can (10 3/4 ounces) condensed cream of chicken soup, undiluted

- 1/4 cup water

PREPARATION

1. In a shallow bowl or food storage bag, combine flour, salt, mustard, paprika, and garlic powder; dredge or toss pork chops to coat well with the seasoned flour mixture. In a skillet over medium heat, brown the chops on both sides in oil. Place pork chops in slow cooker. Combine soup and water; pour over chops. Cover and cook on low for 6 to 8 hours or until meat is tender. If desired, thicken juices and serve with the pork chops.
2. Makes 6 servings.

Chicken, Sausage, and White Bean Chili

INGREDIENTS

- 2 tablespoons extra virgin olive oil

- 2 boneless chicken breast halves, diced

- 12 to 16 ounces chicken sausage, such as chicken apple sausage or chicken other smoked chicken or turkey sausage

- 1 cup chopped onion

- 4 cloves garlic, minced

- 2 cans (about 16 ounces each) Great Northern Beans, drained and rinsed

- 1 1/2 cups tomatillo salsa

- 1 cup chicken broth

- 1 can (14.5 ounces) diced tomatoes with juice, fire-roasted, chili-style, or plain

- 1 cup frozen corn kernels

- 2 tablespoons finely chopped jalapeno peppers, or mild chile peppers

-

1 1/2 teaspoons ground cumin

-

1/2 teaspoon salt

-

1/4 teaspoon ground black pepper

-

Dash cayenne pepper, optional

PREPARATION

1. In a large skillet, heat olive oil over medium heat. Add the onions, diced chicken, and sliced sausage; sauté until onions are tender and chicken is cooked through.
2. Put the drained beans in a 4 to 6-quart slow cooker; add the skillet mixture and all remaining ingredients except cilantro.
3. Cover and cook on HIGH for 3 to 4 hours or LOW for 6 to 8 hours.
4. Sprinkle with cilantro just before serving.
5.

   Serves 6.

Chili Dogs

INGREDIENTS

- 1 pound hot dogs

- 1 large onion, chopped finely

- 2 cans chili with beans (15 oz each)

- 1 teaspoon chili powder

- 4 ounces shredded Cheddar cheese

- hot dog rolls

PREPARATION

1. Combine hot dogs, chopped onion, chili, and chili powder in the slow cooker; stir well.
2. Cover and cook on low for 6 to 9 hours, or high 3 to 4 hours. Spoon sauce over hot dogs in rolls and top each with a little shredded cheese.
3. Serves 6 to 8.

Chinese Style Country Ribs

INGREDIENTS

- 1/4 cup soy sauce

- 1/4 cup orange marmalade

- 1 tablespoon ketchup

- 1 large garlic clove, crushed

- 2 to 3 pounds boneless country-style pork ribs

PREPARATION

1. Combine soy sauce, marmalade, ketchup and garlic.
2. Brush on both sides of the ribs. Place in a slow cooker or crockpot and pour remaining sauce over all.
3. Cover and cook on low for 8 to 10 hours.
4. Serves 6 to 8.

Chinese Crock Pot Dinner

INGREDIENTS

-
1 1/2 pounds pork steak or loin, cut in 1/2-inch strips

-
1 lg. onion, sliced

-
1 sm. green pepper, sliced

-
8 oz. sliced fresh mushrooms

-
1 (8 oz.) can tomato sauce

-
4 carrots, sliced

-
3 tbsp. brown sugar

-
1 1/2 tbsp. vinegar

-
1 1/2 tsp. salt

-
2 tsp. Worcestershire sauce

PREPARATION

1. Brown pork strips in small amount of oil in skillet. Remove excess fat. Place all ingredients with pork in crockpot and cook on low 6 to 8 hours.
2. Serve with hot cooked rice.

Chinese Pork Roast

INGREDIENTS

- 1 pork shoulder roast, about 4 pounds

- 1 teaspoon salt

- 2 teaspoons curry powder

- 2 tablespoons vegetable oil

- 1 can (10 3/4 ounce) condensed cream of mushroom soup or cream of celery soup

- 1/4 cup cold water

- 2 tablespoons all-purpose flour

- 16 ounces frozen Chinese mixed vegetables, cooked until crisp-tender

- 2 cups hot cooked rice

PREPARATION

1. Trim excess fat from roast; cut to fit into crockery cooker, if necessary. Combine salt and 1/2 teaspoon of the curry powder; rub into roast. Brown roast on all sides in hot oil. Place roast on a rack or on a piece of crumpled foil in crockpot. Combine mushroom soup and remaining 1 1/2 teaspoons curry powder; pour over the pork roast. Cover and cook on LOW setting for 8 to 10 hours. Remove roast to a serving platter and keep warm.

2. Pour juices into a saucepan; skim off excess fat. Bring juices to a boil on the stovetop; simmer for 15 minutes. Blend cold water slowly into flour, stirring until smooth; stir into juices. Cook and stir until thickened; serve with hot cooked vegetables, hot cooked rice, and the pork roast.

3. Makes 8 servings.

Choppin' John

INGREDIENTS

- 2 cans (15 oz) black-eyed-peas, drained

- 4 smoked pork chops

- 1 rib celery

- 1 green bell pepper, chopped, or use half green and half red

- 1 large onion, chopped

- 2 cloves garlic, chopped

- 1 teaspoon Worcestershire sauce

- 3 tablespoons brown sugar

- 2 tablespoons ketchup

- 1 jalapeno pepper, chopped, or to taste (optional)

- salt and pepper to taste

PREPARATION

1. Combine all ingredients in the slow cooker/Crock Pot. Cover and cook on low for 6 to 8 hours. Serve over rice with cornbread!
2. Hoppin' John recipe serves 4.

Chutney Pork Loin

INGREDIENTS

- 1 boneless pork loin roast, about 3 to 4 pounds

- 1 large sweet onion, sliced

- Salt and pepper

- 1/2 teaspoon garlic powder or 1 small clove garlic, finely minced

- 1 jar (12 ounces) mango or peach chutney

- 2 tablespoons brown sugar

- 1 tablespoon grainy mustard

- 1/2 teaspoon ground ginger

- 1 teaspoon curry powder

PREPARATION

1. Wash roast and pat dry; trim excess fat.
2. Put sliced onion in the bottom of a 5 to 7-quart slow cooker. Lightly salt and pepper the roast then rub with the garlic powder or fresh minced garlic. Place the roast in the slow cooker. Combine remaining ingredients and spoon over the roast. Cover and cook on HIGH for 1 hour, then reduce to LOW and cook for 6 to 8 hours longer, or continue cooking on HIGH for 3 to 4 hours longer.
3. The roast should register at least 160° on an instant read thermometer or meat thermometer inserted in the center of the roast.
4. Remove the roast from the crockpot and keep warm; pour juices into a medium saucepan. Simmer the juices for about 5 to 8 minutes to reduce by about one-third. Combine 1 tablespoon cornstarch with 1 tablespoon cold water, stirring until smooth. Stir the cornstarch mixture into the juices and continue cooking for about 1 minute, until thickened.
5. Serves 6 to 8.

Cider Pork Pot Roast

INGREDIENTS

- 2 medium onions, halved and sliced

- 1 boneless pork shoulder or sirloin roast, about 3 1/2 to 4 1/2 pounds

- 4 to 6 carrots, cut in 1-inch pieces

- 2 cloves garlic, minced

- 1/2 teaspoon salt

- 1/8 teaspoon pepper

- 1/2 teaspoon allspice

- 1 teaspoon chili powder

- 1 teaspoon dried leaf marjoram or thyme

- 2 cups natural apple juice or cider

- 2 tablespoons cider vinegar

PREPARATION

1. Arrange onions in the bottom of the slow cooker.
2. Leave netting on pork roast and place in the slow cooker.
3. Arrange carrots around the roast; sprinkle the roast with the garlic, salt, pepper, allspice, chili powder, and marjoram or thyme. Combine the juice and vinegar and pour over the roast.
4. Cover and cook on HIGH for 1 hour. Reduce heat to LOW and cook for 6 to 8 hours longer, or leave on HIGH for 3 to 4 hours longer.
5. Pour juices into a saucepan and bring to a boil on the stovetop. Reduce to medium and continue boiling for 5 minutes.
6. Combine flour and cold water until smooth; whisk into the simmering juices. Continue cooking and stirring until thickened. Serve with the pork.
7. Serves 6 to 8.

Cider-Sweet Ham

INGREDIENTS

- 1 fully cooked ham, about 3 pounds

- 4 cups (32 ounces) apple cider or apple juice

- 2 teaspoons dry mustard

- 1 cup brown sugar, firmly packed

- 1/2 teaspoon ground cloves

- 1/4 teaspoon allspice

- dash nutmeg

- 2 cups golden raisins

PREPARATION

1. Place ham with enough cider to cover into your slow cooker/Crock Pot and cook on low for 10 to 12 hours.

Confetti Mac 'n Cheese with Ham

INGREDIENTS

- 1 center-cut ham slice, about 12 to 16 ounces, diced

- 1 rib celery, chopped

- 1 tablespoon minced dried onion, or use chopped fresh onion

- 2 teaspoons dried parsley

- 1 teaspoon celery seed

- 1 package (8 ounces)Kraft® Classic Melts Cheddar-American shredded cheese or an American process cheese

- 1 can (10 3/4 oz) condensed cream of celery soup, undiluted

- 1 can diced tomatoes with juice

- 1 cup frozen mixed vegetables (peas, carrots, green beans), thawed

- black pepper to taste

- 5 to 6 cups hot, cooked macaroni

PREPARATION

1. Combine all ingredients, except mixed vegetables and macaroni, in the slow cooker or crockpot. Cover and cook on low for 6 to 7 hours. Add vegetables about 1 hour before serving (or microwave them and add just before serving). Cook macaroni until just tender; drain. Pour crockpot mixture into a large serving bowl. Mix in macaroni (a little less than the full amount if you like it very saucy).
2. Crockpot macaroni and cheese recipe serves 4 to 6.

Corn and Ham Crockpot

INGREDIENTS

- 3 cups frozen whole kernel corn, thawed

- 1 1/2 cups diced lean ham

- 1/2 cup finely chopped onion

- 1/4 cup chopped green onion

- 1/2 cup chopped green bell pepper or red bell pepper or combination

- 1 can (10 3/4 ounces) condensed cream of mushroom soup

- 1/8 teaspoon ground black pepper

- 3/4 cup shredded Cheddar cheese

PREPARATION

1. Spray liner of crockpot with cooking spray or lightly rub with oil. In crockpot, combine the corn, ham, onion and green onion, green pepper, mushroom soup, and pepper. Stir in Cheddar cheese. Cover and cook on LOW for 4 1/2 to 6 hours.
2. Serves 4 to 6.

Corn, Ham and Potato Scallop

INGREDIENTS

- 6 cups peeled baking potatoes, cut in 1-inch cubes

- 1 1/2 cups diced cooked ham, beef, or other leftover meat or poultry

- 1 to 1 1/2 cups whole kernel corn, from can or frozen thawed

- 1/4 cup finely chopped green bell pepper

- 1/4 cup finely chopped onion

- 1 can (10 3/4 ounces) condensed Cheddar cheese soup

- 1/2 cup milk

- 2 tablespoons all-purpose flour

PREPARATION

1. In slow cooker, combine sliced potatoes, ham, corn, bell pepper and onion; stir to mix well.
2. In small bowl, combine soup, milk and flour; whisk until smooth. Pour soup mixture over vegetable mixture; carefully stir to blend.
3. Cover and cook on LOW for 7 to 9 hours, or until potatoes are tender.

Corn-Stuffed Pork Chops

INGREDIENTS

- 6 thick pork chops, 1 to 2 inches thick

- 3/4 cup thawed frozen corn kernels, or use canned, drained

- 1 cup soft bread crumbs

- 1 teaspoon onion, minced

- 2 tablespoons green bell pepper, chopped

- 1 teaspoon salt

- 1/2 teaspoon crumbled dried leaf sage

PREPARATION

1. With a sharp knife cut a horizontal slit in the side of each chop forming a pocket for stuffing. Mix undrained corn, bread crumbs, onion, pepper, salt, and sage. Spoon corn mixture into the slits. Secure with toothpicks or small skewers. Place on a metal rack or trivet in crockpot. Or, crumple a piece of aluminum foil to form a makeshift rack. Cover and cook on LOW for 6 to 8 hours, until pork is tender.
2. Makes 4 to 6 servings.

Country Pork with Mushrooms

INGREDIENTS

- 2 pounds country-style ribs, boneless

- 1 can cream of mushrooms soup

- 4 ounces sliced mushrooms

- 1/4 teaspoon salt

- 1 envelope mushroom gravy mix

- 1/8 teaspoon pepper

- 1/2 teaspoon sweet paprika

- 2 tablespoons cold water blended with 1 heaping tablespoon all-purpose flour

PREPARATION

1. Combine boneless ribs, soup, mushrooms, salt, pepper, gravy, and paprika in crockpot. Cover and cook on LOW setting for 7 to 9 hours. Stir flour mixture into broth and cook on HIGH heat setting an additional 15 minutes, or until thickened. Serve country-style ribs with mashed potatoes and corn.
2. Country-style ribs recipe serves 6.

Country-Style Ribs & Sauerkraut

INGREDIENTS

- 1 bag sauerkraut, rinsed & drained

- 1 onion

- 1 red-skinned apple

- 2 to 3 pounds country style pork ribs

- 1 cup beer

PREPARATION

1. Put sauerkraut in bottom of slow cooker/Crock Pot. Add diced onion and chopped apple. Do not need to peel apple. Stir and even top. Layer country ribs on top of kraut mixture. Pour beer over all. Cover and cook on low from 8 to 10 hours.
2. Serves 4 to 6.

Country Pork with Mushrooms

INGREDIENTS

- 2 pounds country-style ribs, boneless

- 1 can cream of mushrooms soup

- 4 ounces sliced mushrooms

- 1/4 teaspoon salt

- 1 envelope mushroom gravy mix

- 1/8 teaspoon pepper

- 1/2 teaspoon sweet paprika

- 2 tablespoons cold water blended with 1 heaping tablespoon all-purpose flour

PREPARATION

1. Combine boneless ribs, soup, mushrooms, salt, pepper, gravy, and paprika in crockpot. Cover and cook on LOW setting for 7 to 9 hours. Stir flour mixture into broth and cook on HIGH heat setting an additional 15 minutes, or until thickened. Serve country-style ribs with mashed potatoes and corn.
2. Country-style ribs recipe serves 6.

Cranberry-Apple Pork Ribs

INGREDIENTS

- 2 cups cranberries (8 ounces)

- 1/3 cup maple syrup

- 1/3 cup packed brown sugar

- 1/2 cup water

- 1 Granny Smith apple, diced, about 1 cup

- 1 teaspoon Dijon mustard

- 1/4 teaspoon cinnamon

- 1/4 teaspoon mace or nutmeg

- 3 to 4 pounds boneless country style ribs

- 1 bag (16 ounces) frozen small white onions, or 1 large onions, sliced

- 1 tablespoon cornstarch mixed with 1 to 2 tablespoons cold water, optional•

PREPARATION

1. In a saucepan, combine the cranberries, syrup, brown sugar, water, and apple; bring to a boil. Reduce heat to medium-low and simmer for 5 minutes. Stir in mustard, cinnamon, and mace or nutmeg.
2. Arrange onions in the bottom of the crockery insert of a 5 to 7-quart slow cooker. Put pork ribs on top of the onions then spoon the cranberry sauce evenly over all. Cover and cook on LOW for 7 to 9 hours, until pork is tender.
3. Serves 6 to 8.

Cran-Apple Pork Roast

INGREDIENTS

-
1 (3 to 4 lb) boneless pork loin roast

-
2 cloves garlic, minced

-
1 can whole cranberry sauce

-
1/4 c brown sugar

-
1/2 c apple juice

-
2 apples, cored, peeled and coarsely chopped

-
salt and pepper to taste

PREPARATION

1. Place roast in slow cooker; rub all over with the minced garlic. Add remaining ingredients and cook on low for 7 to 9 hours. Pork should be about 160° when fully cooked. Serve with rice.
2. Serves 4 to 6.

Cranberry Pork Roast

INGREDIENTS

- 1 boneless rolled pork loin roast

- 1 can (16-oz.) jellied or whole berry cranberry sauce

- 1/2 cup granulated sugar

- 1/4 cup cranberry juice

- 1 teaspoon dry mustard

- 1/4 teaspoon ground cloves

- 2 tablespoons cornstarch

- 2 tablespoons cold water

- salt

PREPARATION

1. Place pork loin roast in slow cooker. In a medium bowl, mash cranberry sauce; stir in sugar, cranberry juice, mustard, and cloves. Pour over roast. Cover crockpot and cook on low for 6 to 8 hours, or until pork roast is tender.

Pork should register about 155 to 160° when done. Remove pork roast and keep warm.
2. Skim fat from juices; measure 2 cups -- add water if necessary -- and pour into a saucepan.
3. Bring to a boil over medium high heat.
4. Combine the cornstarch and cold water until smooth; stir into gravy. Continue to cook, stirring, until thickened. Season with salt and serve with sliced pork roast.

This pork is delicious with rice, or serve with seasoned stuffing and potatoes.

Creamy Ham and Broccoli

INGREDIENTS

- 1/2 cup. chopped onion

- 3 cups chopped ham, or use cooked chopped chicken or turkey

- 16 oz. frozen cut broccoli, thawed

- 1 can condensed cream of mushroom soup

- 1 jar (8 oz.) pasteurized process cheese spread

- 1 can (8 oz.) sliced water chestnuts, drained

- 1 cup. uncooked converted rice

- 1/2 cup water

- 1/2 cup milk

- 1/2 cup. chopped celery

- 1/2 tsp. pepper

- paprika (optional)

PREPARATION

1. In slow cooker, combine ham, broccoli, soup, cheese spread, water chestnuts, rice, milk, celery, onion and pepper. Stir until blended. Smooth top, pushing rice into mixture. Cover and cook on high for 2 - 2 1/2 hours or on low for 4-5 hours or until rice and onion are tender, stirring occasionally if possible. Check near end of cooking time to make sure the rice does not get too mushy.

Creamy Pork

INGREDIENTS

- 1/2 cup chopped onion

- 3 cloves garlic, minced, or 3/4 teaspoon garlic powder

- 2 Granny Smith apples, peeled, cored and sliced

- 2 teaspoons sugar

- 1/2 teaspoon dried leaf sage, crumbled

- 1/4 teaspoon ground nutmeg

- 1/8 teaspoon pepper

- 2 to 3 pounds boneless pork loin, trimmed and cut into 1-inch cubes

- 1/4 cup all-purpose flour

- 1/2 cup dry white wine

- 1 tablespoon plus 2 teaspoons cornstarch

- 1/3 cup whipping cream

- salt to taste

PREPARATION

1. In slow cooker combine chopped onion, garlic, apples, sugar, sage, and pepper. Coat pork cubes with flour and add to slow cooker. Pour in wine. Cover and cook on LOW for 7 to 9 hours. In a small bowl, whisk together the cornstarch and whipping cream. Turn slow cooker to HIGH and pour into pork mixture; cook for 15 to 20 minutes longer. Season to taste with salt. Serve with cornmeal biscuits or cornbread.

Creamy Pork Tenderloin w/Veggies

INGREDIENTS

- 1 1/2 to 2 pounds pork tenderloin

- 1 small head cabbage, coarsely chopped

- 1 medium onion, chopped

- 1 envelope stroganoff seasoning

- 1 envelope mushroom gravy

- 1 can cream of celery soup

- 1/4 cup water

- 1 teaspoon caraway seed

- pepper to taste

- 1 to 2 cups frozen green beans

- 1/3 cup half-and-half

PREPARATION

1. Cut pork into 1-inch cubes; place in 3 1/2-quart or larger slow cooker. Add onion and cabbage. Combine stroganoff mix, gravy mix, soup, water, caraway seed and pepper together; pour over pork mixture and stir to coat. Cover and cook on low 7 to 9 hours. About 30 minutes before serving, turn to high and add frozen green beans. Add half and half just before serving. Delicious over noodles or served with biscuits.
2. Serves 6.

Creamy Shells with Ham & Smoked Cheese

INGREDIENTS

- 12 ounces diced ham

- 1 can cream of celery soup

- 8 ounces smoked Gouda cheese

- black pepper to taste

- 1 cup frozen vegetables, cut broccoli or mixed

- 3 cups cooked small pasta shells or macaroni

- 1/4 cup of evaporated milk, low fat

PREPARATION

1. In a crockpot, 3 1/2-quart to 5-quart, combine ham, soup, cheese, and pepper. Cover and cook on low for 4 to 5 hours. Add frozen vegetables 30 minutes before serving. Add milk to thin; add hot cooked pasta then serve.
2. Creamy shells with ham and cheese recipe serves 4.

Creole Chicken With Sausage

INGREDIENTS

-

1 1/2 pounds boneless chicken thighs, cut into chunks

-

12 ounces smoked andouille sausage, cut in 1- to 2-inch lengths

-

1 cup chopped onions

-

3/4 cup chicken broth or water

-

1 can (14.5 ounces) diced tomatoes

-

1 can (6 ounces) tomato paste

-

2 teaspoons Cajun or Creole seasoning

-

dash cayenne pepper, to taste

-

1 green bell pepper, chopped

-

salt and pepper, to taste

-

hot cooked white or brown rice or cooked drained spaghetti

PREPARATION

1. In a slow cooker, combine the chicken thigh pieces, andouille sausage pieces, chopped onions, broth or water, tomatoes (with their juices), tomato paste, Creole seasoning, and cayenne pepper.
2. Cover and cook the chicken and sausage mixture on LOW for 6 to 7 hours. Add the chopped green bell pepper about an hour before the dish is done. Taste and add salt and pepper, as needed.
3. Serve this flavorful chicken and sausage dish over hot boiled rice, or serve it with spaghetti or angel hair pasta.
4. Serves 6.

Crockery Ham

INGREDIENTS

- 1 fully cooked ham, about 5 to 7 pounds (with or without the bone, butt or shank half)

- whole cloves

- 1/2 cup currant jelly

- 1 tablespoon vinegar

- 1/2 teaspoon dry mustard

- 1/2 teaspoon ground cinnamon

PREPARATION

1. Place a metal rack or trivet (or crumpled foil "rack") in the crockpot and place ham on it. Cover and cook on low 5 to 6 hours. Remove ham and pour off juices; remove skin and fat. Score ham and stud with the whole cloves. In a small saucepan, melt jelly with vinegar, mustard and cinnamon. Remove metal rack or trivet. Return ham to crockpot and spoon sauce over scored ham. Cover and cook on high for 20 to 30 minutes, brushing with sauce from time to time.
2. Slice and serve ham hot or cold.

Crock Pot Carnitas

INGREDIENTS

- 2 to 4 lb. pork shoulder roast

- 4 garlic cloves, peeled, each clove cut into 4 pieces

- 1 fresh jalapeno pepper

- 1 bunch fresh cilantro

- 1 can beer (12 ounces)

- Corn tortillas

PREPARATION

1. With a knife, cut several small slits into the roast. Insert pieces of garlic cloves in roast; place in crockpot with whole pepper and half bunch of cilantro which has been chopped. Season to taste. Pour in beer. Cook on HIGH 4 to 6 hours until fork tender (LOW 9 to 11 hours). Remove meat; shred. Serve with warm tortillas, with by your choice of garnishes. Suggested garnishes: diced tomatoes, onions, sliced ripe olives, shredded lettuce, sour cream, cheese, salsa, guacamole, and cilantro.

Crock Pot Chops Or Ribs

INGREDIENTS

-

6 or 8 pork chops, or cut up spareribs to nearly fill slow cooker

-

.

-

Sauce

-

1/4 cup chopped onion

-

1/2 cup chopped celery

-

1 cup ketchup

-

1/2 cup water

-

1/4 cup lemon juice

-

2 tbsp. brown sugar

-

2 tbsp. Worcestershire sauce

-

2 tbsp. vinegar

-

1 tbsp. mustard

-

1/2 tsp. salt

-

1/4 tsp. pepper

PREPARATION

1. If using spareribs, boil or roast them for about 30 minutes to eliminate some of the excess fat. Drain and put in crockpot.
2. Mix together sauce ingredients and pour over chops or ribs in pot. Cook for 8 to 10 hours, until tender. Serve with hot cooked rice or potatoes.
3. Serves 6.

Crockpot Cola Ham

INGREDIENTS

- 1/2 cup brown sugar

- 1 tsp dry mustard

- 1/4 cup cola (Coca Cola, Dr. Pepper, etc.)

- 3 to 4 pound pre-cooked ham

PREPARATION

1. Combine brown sugar and mustard. Moisten with just enough cola to make a smooth paste. Reserve remaining cola. Score the ham with shallow slashes in a diamond pattern. Rub ham with paste mixture. Place ham in slow cooker/Crock Pot and add remaining cola. Cover and cook on high for 1 hour, then turn to low and cook for 6 to 7 hours.
2. Serves 9 to 12.
3. A 5 pound ham could be cooked in a larger slow cooker.
4. Cook for 1 hour on high, then 8 to 10 hours on low.

Crock Pot Glorified Pork Chops

INGREDIENTS

-

6 Pork Chops (comes out to about 1.5 pounds or so but you can do more or less to your needs)

-

1 Medium onion sliced (1/2 Cup)

-

1 Can (10-3/4 oz.) Condensed cream of celery soup

-

1/4 C. water

-

pepper, to taste

-

dry boxed stuffing mix,

PREPARATION

1. Place chops in crockpot. Cover with sliced onions, condensed soup (directly from the can) and 1/4 cup water. Add pepper to taste. Cover and cook all day (7 to 8 hours) on LOW or 1/2 Day (3 to 4 hours) on HIGH in crockpot. You can also add a package of dry boxed stuffing (with herb packet) on top of chops first then the onions and soup and water.
2. Unbelievably moist, tender chops.

Crock Pot Ham

INGREDIENTS

- 1 small ham

- apple juice to cover

- 1 cup brown sugar

- 2 tsp. dry mustard

- 1 tsp. ground cloves

- 2 cup raisins

PREPARATION

1. Cook ham in juice 8-10 hours on low. Before serving turn oven to 375 degrees. Make a paste of the sugar, mustard, cloves and about 1 tablespoon of the hot juice. Smear on ham. Place ham in a baking pan and pour in a cup full of the hot juice and the raisins. Bake 30 minutes or until the paste has turned into a glaze.

Crockpot Ham And Potatoes

INGREDIENTS

- 6 to 8 slices ham, deli sliced or from leftover ham, about 1/8-inch thick

- 8 to 10 medium potatoes, peeled and thinly sliced

- 1 med. onion, peeled and thinly sliced

- salt and pepper

- 1 1/2 cups grated Cheddar cheese

- 2 cans condensed cream of celery or cream of mushroom soup

- paprika

PREPARATION

1. Put half of ham, potatoes and onions in Crock Pot. Sprinkle with salt and pepper, then 1 cup of the grated cheese. Add remaining ham, potatoes and onions, and spoon undiluted soup over the top. Sprinkle with remaining 1/2 cup cheese and paprika.
2. Cover and cook on low for 8 hours or on high 4 hours.

Crockpot Ham Tetrazzini

INGREDIENTS

-

1 can (10 3/4 ounces) condensed cream of celery soup

-

1/2 cup evaporated milk

-

1/2 cup grated Parmesan cheese

-

1 1/2 cups cubed cooked ham

-

8 ounces sliced mushrooms, sautéed in a little butter

-

1/4 cup dry white wine

-

1 small package spaghetti, (5 oz)

-

2 tablespoons butter, melted

-

Parmesan cheese

PREPARATION

1. Combine all ingredients except spaghetti and butter in slow cooker; stir well. Cover and cook on LOW setting for 6 to 8 hours.
2. Just before serving, cook spaghetti according to package directions; drain and toss with butter. Stir into ham mixture in slow cooker. Sprinkle additional grated Parmesan cheese just before serving.
3. Serves 4.

CPSIA information can be obtained
at www.ICGtesting.com
Printed in the USA
BVHW050629160522
637110BV00014B/298